The GP Trainer's Handbook

an educational guide for trainers by trainers

Second Edition

Paul Middleton
BM(Hons), MA (Education), FRCGP, DRCOG

and

Maurice Price
MBBS, DRCOG, MRCGP

Foreword by
Steve Field
CBE, FRCP, FRCGP
Chairman
Royal College of General Practitioners

Radcliffe Publishing
London • New York

Radcliffe Publishing Ltd
33–41 Dallington Street
London
EC1V 0BB
United Kingdom

www.radcliffepublishing.com

Electronic catalogue and worldwide online ordering facility.

First Edition 2001

British Library Cataloguing in Publication Data

A catalogue record for this book is available from the British Library.

ISBN-13: 978 184619 423 8

The paper used for the text pages of this book is FSC® certified. FSC® (The Forest Stewardship Council) is an international network to promote responsible management of the world's forests.

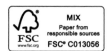

Typeset by Phoenix Photosetting, Chatham, Kent
Printed and bound by TJI Digital, Padstow, Cornwall

Contents

Web-based resources

The following resources referred to in the text can be downloaded from www.radcliffepublishing.com/gptrainershandbook

1 **Bare essentials: how do you become a trainer?**
Criteria for becoming a training practice

2 **Induction: how do trainers settle a trainee into the practice?**
Appointment form
Model contract
Educational philosophy agreement
Useful telephone numbers
Maslow's scale and educational needs hierarchy

3 **Assessment of learning: how do trainers assess learning needs?**
GP clinical strategies form
Statistical terms
Critical appraisal
READER
The 19-point guide to educational supervision
The friendly guide to the e-portfolio and ARCP
Initial educational planning form
Initial assessment grid
Skills checklist
Assessment of attitudinal needs

4 **The e-portfolio and other curricular tools: how do trainers use curricular tools?**
Personal development plan assessment tool
Need to know list
Forms you should know
The Wolverhampton grid

5 **Tutorials: how do trainers plan tutorials?**
Hemispheric dominance indicator
VAK indicator
Field dependence model

About the authors

Paul Middleton joined his rural practice in 1987 after six years in the RAF and became a GP trainer in 1989. He has been actively involved with undergraduate and postgraduate training ever since and completed an MA in Education at Bath University in 2007.

Paul has a fervent belief in the bottom-up approach to training and this had been constantly reinforced by meeting other trainers and trainees. The first *GP Trainer's Handbook* published in 2001 aimed to capture this wisdom – and this manual has repeated that process in a training terrain that has changed dramatically.

Maurice Price joined his town practice in 2007 and was one of the youngest postgraduate course organisers to be appointed in 2005. He completed his Certificate of Medical Education at Stafford University in 2005.

Maurice is the 'Tigger' of the team, bouncing with enthusiasm and encouragement. He has found teaching to be one of the greatest ways to nourish his own development, as well as those around him.

Foreword

The first edition of *The GP Trainer's Handbook* was a project that Paul and I co-ordinated with the support of many GP trainers from across the West Midlands. We received lots of positive feedback and many ideas and suggestions. It has become a hugely successful resource for GP trainers and programme directors in the UK and indeed across the world.

The last 10 years has ushered in major changes to GP training and as Chairman of the Royal College of General Practitioners, I have had a ring-side view! I am really pleased that the RCGP's Curriculum for GP Training was approved without amendment by the regulator and that it has been successfully rolled out across the country. I know that the MRCGP is among the best medical assessments in the world and I am pleased that trainees spend a greater proportion of their training in general practice.

Trainers have adapted superbly to the demands of these changes. I am delighted with their innovative and stimulating contributions and that Paul and Maurice have found the time and energy to produce this excellent second edition which is a testament to their ingenuity and flexibility.

The next generation of GPs will face even more changes in the landscape of primary care and it has become even more imperative that we provide high-quality training. This manual will support this process.

Professor Steve Field CBE, FRCP, FRCGP
GP, Bellevue Medical Centre, Birmingham
Chairman of Council, RCGP 2007-2010
Chairman, National Health Inclusion Board
January 2011

Preface

THE NOUGHTY CHANGES

Ten years ago, trainers in the West Midlands collaborated to produce a 'bottom-up' trainer's guide to training. This process has been repeated in a very different training environment – so what has changed? It might be easier to say what hasn't changed – and this is perhaps the focus of this book because about the only aspect of training that hasn't been revolutionised is the one-to-one relationship that exists between trainer and trainee. This is the lynch pin of training and the aim of this manual is to help these two central players to tackle the challenge of GP training together.

So what has changed? Let's borrow Donabedian's classification to look at this:

➤ **Structural change:** VTS programmes have now have a different classification (ST1, 2, 3) for trainees who often come out to practices much earlier in training. Trainers can have many hats too – with educational supervisor (ES) and clinical supervisor (CS) roles.
➤ We now have the new curriculum, Workplace-based assessment (WPBA), a 'New MRCGP' – MRCGP for a while – the thankful disappearance of summative assessment along with the emergence of the e-portfolio and a lot of new acronyms (DOPS, Minicex, CbD, ARCPs, AiTs).
➤ Trainers are now much more likely to have studied/be studying for one of the many educational qualifications on offer.
➤ Training practices are much more likely to have medical students, foundation doctors, nursing students, more than one GP trainee and more than one trainer – and probably in the same premises, now creaking at the seams!
➤ The internet was a footnote (albeit a fair sized one) 10 years ago, and now
. . .
➤ **Process:** trainers now have an over-arching system of training through which they have to navigate with their trainee. We live in the world of competence and trainees now have to demonstrate this in a number of environments (WPBA in primary and secondary care, the MRCGP, Clinical Skills Assessment (CSA) and Applied Knowledge Test (AKT)). Trainers undertake roles in supervision and assessment. Adult learning may not

have changed, but the systems that guide this process in general practice have.

➤ **Outcomes:** trainees now face only one assessment system but they have to demonstrate competent performance against a large number of defined criteria, they have to pass the MRCGP and they have to satisfy an Annual Review of Competence Progression (ARCP). Trainer performance is not yet scrutinised to the same degree but quality of teaching and training remains an important issue.

General practice is itself in a different place too – the concept of professionalism has altered and our relationship with society has evolved. We are arguably no longer perceived as the 'expert' who can be trusted and deferred to – we are perhaps now the 'partner' who must prove (and keep proving) worthy of the role. This is the changing world we are preparing our trainees for.

So where does this book fit in? It aims to provide a tool-box of resources, with advice on where and when to use the tools and where to get help if you need it. Hippocrates wrote 2000 years ago that it was a doctor's duty 'to give a share of precepts and oral instruction and all the other learning to . . . pupils who have signed the covenant and have taken the oath according to medical law'. Despite the absence of a similar clause in the GMC 'Duties of a Doctor', we feel it still remains a duty, a privilege and a pleasure (usually!) to be involved in the training of the next generation of our colleagues. If this manual adds even a little to the process, we will feel it has succeeded in its aims.

Paul Middleton
Maurice Price
January 2011

CHAPTER 1

Bare essentials: how do you become a trainer?

WHY DO YOU WANT TO BE A TRAINER?

Becoming a GP trainer can be one of the most challenging and rewarding experiences throughout your career. The presence of a trainee often acts as a catalyst for your own personal development. Brown (1999) discusses some of the motivations for becoming a trainer. The decision to become a trainer is often taken on an individual basis. However, we must keep in mind how this will impact on the practice. The decision to become a training practice must involve the practice as a whole. It is worth considering the following points.

1   Why are we considering training? Challenge, money, more doctor time?
2   How will we all contribute to the process? Do we all *want* to contribute?
3   Do we appreciate the time commitments, especially time out of the practice for the trainer?
4   Are their financial considerations, e.g. purchasing equipment, missed opportunities for adding quality outcomes framework (QOF) data in the early days of seeing patients?
5   What do we feel about a 'trainee' doctor seeing our patients? How will the patients feel?

Ensure that you discuss these issues with all doctors in the practice. Those with little or no experience of training may feel quite threatened by the thought of a trainee. The more they are involved the better. It will de-mystify the process, and you will often find they rather enjoy giving sessions like tutorials, especially when they realise they *do* seem to know more than the trainee!

In summary – ensure you know what you, your colleagues and the practice are letting yourselves in for!

THE APPROVAL PROCESS

Applying to become a trainer and getting approved means hoops to be jumped through and also a reasonable amount of paperwork. There is no way to make this section sexy, so here goes!

Postgraduate training in general practice is regulated by the Postgraduate Medical Education and Training Board (PMETB). The PMETB is legally responsible for the approval of all general practice training posts and assessing applications for and issuing certificates of completion of training (CCT), without which it is not possible to work as a general practitioner in the UK.

The PMETB has devolved the responsibility of approving all training posts for general practice both in hospital and in training practices to the Postgraduate School of General Practice (PSGP), which selects suitable GP trainers and recommends approval to the PMETB. The PSGP is responsible for establishing relevant local criteria for the selection of trainers, at the same time as ensuring that the PMETB national criteria for training standards are also met in full. Depending on which area you work in, the responsibilities may be further devolved to directors looking after your local area.

There will be some variation between deaneries on the actual approval process and criteria that need to be met. The following link shows the criteria for selection of general practice trainers in the West Midlands Deanery: www. westmidlandsdeanery.nhs.uk/LinkClick.aspx?fileticket=3fEmDqevZ2c%3d&tabid=167&mid=896

Similar criteria will be available either from your deanery website or by contacting them directly. These requirements and processes can feel quite daunting, so here is a summary of the general principals for becoming a trainer, which will be pretty consistent between deaneries.

To become a GP trainer, a GP must:
➤ satisfactorily complete an approved course in general practice training
➤ fulfil the requirements laid down in the deanery's document
➤ subsequently apply to become a GP trainer
➤ undergo a practice visit.

Courses will vary between deaneries; they can be modular running over a number of sessions through the year, or a week-long residential course. There is now an expectation that this will become a 'Certificate of Medical Education' although this is not yet compulsory. Details of available trainers' courses can be found by contacting your local deanery. The following links relate to generic courses in medical education such as the Certificate of Medical Education:
➤ www.dundee.ac.uk/meded/frames/home.html (distance learning opportunity to achieve Certificate in Medical Education)
➤ www.staffs.ac.uk/study_here/courses/medical-education-tcm429808.jsp (face-to-face modular course to achieve Certificate in Medical Education)
➤ www.scalingtheheights.com/ (courses often aimed at those with experience in teaching to 'expand their horizons').

The criteria for training approval look at both the trainer and the resources (i.e. the practice) in which the training will take place. Expectations for a trainer will include:

➤ will have at least three years experience in general practice following completion of their vocational training
➤ be members of the Royal College of General Practitioners (RCGP) (although there are alternatives to this)
➤ must have up-to-date equality and diversity training
➤ should participate in their deanery selection process for GP trainees
➤ have regular attendance at their local educators' group
➤ will have completed an approved trainer's course.

Expectations for the practice will include the following:

➤ must normally have achieved the maximum QOF points for medical records
➤ GP specialty training registrars (GPStRs) must consult in a well-equipped room that meets local deanery standards
➤ GPStRs should have their own space and facilities in the practice to secure personal items safely
➤ IT support must be available in the practice, including a computer with appropriate search facilities, internet and electronic reference access, as well as facilities for private study
➤ the list size and workload of the practice must be large enough to offer GPStRs a wide variety of clinical experience representing normal, everyday general practice
➤ have up-to-date and effective policies for home visiting, continuity of care for patients, emergency care and out-of-hours cover
➤ manage an active programme of audit that demonstrates the full audit cycle, and the application of both standards and criteria
➤ undertake regular significant event analysis
➤ have regular practice meetings, which the GPStR is expected to attend and at which practice management and the management of patients are discussed.

Again, an example of a deanery's full list of criteria can be found at: www.westmidlandsdeanery.nhs.uk/LinkClick.aspx?fileticket=3fEmDqevZ2c%3d&tabid=167&mid=896

Although this looks quite daunting, let's read between the lines. What they are looking for is an up-to-date, enthusiastic trainer who is willing to maintain his or her own personal development in relation to training. In relation to the practice it requires a well-performing practice with adequate space/resources and an ability to review its performance and respond to these findings. Most practices are doing this to some degree anyway, much of this links in with QOF requirements and this will look impressive on your next appraisal.

Remember that each deanery may have a slightly different system/adapted criteria so it is important that you obtain this. This has hopefully given you an idea of the sort of expectations they will have for you and your practice.

ATTRACTING A TRAINEE

Chapter 2 discusses the current process for trainees entering GP training. Trainees are now either allocated to practices from their local scheme or are given a time frame in which to choose. Either way, you will still want to 'market' yourself to become an attractive practice to potential trainees.

So what are trainees looking for? The following is an anecdote from a recently attended evening at the local education centre. Trainers were 'marketing' themselves and their practice to potential trainees. Trainers prepared themselves with information such as list size, recent pass rates and skills available from the doctors within the practice. Once their brief presentation had finished, the first question from nearly every trainee was 'Thank you, so how many miles are you from Birmingham? How long will it take me to get there?' Location, location, location will always be an issue for trainees and obviously we can't change our location! On-call commitment is currently not as big an issue, due to the loss of out-of-hours responsibility (although watch this space...). So what can you use to make yourself more attractive to potential trainees? Points to consider include the following.

➤ If you are a new training practice, consider attending your local half-day release training programme. This allows you to meet the trainees and also allows you to get a better idea of the teaching they are part of.

➤ Does your local course have a 'meet the trainers' day for local practices? If not, it may be worth asking if one can be arranged.

➤ Everything nowadays exists in 'cyberspace'. How up to date is your website? Does it have a specific trainee section? Does it have useful links for training? Is the information on your local vocational training scheme (VTS) website accurate and up to date?

➤ What can you offer that may make you more unique? Acupuncture, doctors with special interests, maybe one of you is an MRCGP examiner?

➤ Can you get feedback from previous trainees to show to current trainees? Even if you don't do this formally, they will ask through the grapevine.

➤ Attend your local GP trainer's workshop; they will give you an opinion on what the current generation of trainees are looking for.

SUMMARY

The process for becoming a trainer in a training practice can feel hugely daunting. However, many of the practice requirements will already be in place and ultimately having a trainee on board will enhance the careers of both you and your colleagues. Happy hunting . . .

Induction: how do trainers settle a trainee into the practice?

Sit down and have some tea said the Mad Hatter
(Lewis Carroll, *Alice in Wonderland*)

INTRODUCTION

I can remember feeling just like Alice at the Mad Hatter's party when I arrived in general practice. Here I was after years of training, raring to go. But patients kept describing things that baffled me, and that was when they *were* ill – most of them hadn't even got the good grace to have an illness at all! I was either

Table 2.1 Maslow's hierarchy of human needs

SELF-ACTUALISATION
realisation of innate potential
self-expression
self-fulfilment
self-respect
self-confidence

ESTEEM NEEDS
esteem
status
approval

BELONGINGNESS NEEDS
love
intimacy
acknowledgement

SAFETY NEEDS
boundaries
predictability
stability

PHYSIOLOGICAL NEEDS
sleep
sex
food/drink, etc.

mad or the rules had changed – like Alice, I discovered the latter was true. Sadly, this still appears to be true to a degree today. So what do trainers do about it?

Maslow's (1972) hierarchy of human needs is one method of looking at this problem. Neighbour (1992) develops this concept into the hierarchy of educational perspectives. These hierarchies are shown in Tables 2.1 and 2.2.

Table 2.2 Hierarchy of educational needs

AUTONOMY
takes responsibility for own learning
successfully evolves from trainee to principal
sense of purpose, worth and direction

SELF-ESTEEM
uses self in consultation
achieved a balanced lifestyle
tolerates uncertainty, occasional mistakes
knows limitations
can challenge accepted wisdom/trainer

RECOGNITION
hungry for new ideas
interested in the wider sphere of primary care
can accept praise/criticism
confidence growing independent of trainer

CONFIDENCE
accepted in primary health care team (PHCT)
uses and contributes to PHCT
bonds with trainer
sees wider scope of spectrum of illness

SAFETY
able and willing to ask for help
knows where to access resources
basic clinical skills and knowledge

SURVIVAL
knows timetable
satisfactory environment
working knowledge of admin system (phones, paperwork, geography services, etc.)
free enough from non-medical worries

These lists can be used to develop an introductory programme that allows trainees to feel their way into general practice. Maslow's scale is now considered flawed (when did you last get out of bed because your self-esteem was calling? and what does 'self-actualisation' actually mean? The answer being that: if you have to ask, you don't have it!). Figure 2.1 illustrates a more accepted model

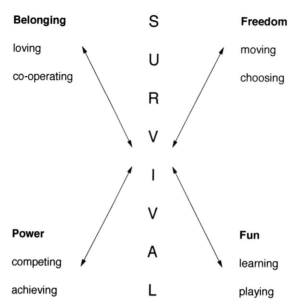

Figure 2.1: Glasser's motivating factors.

of human needs based on survival (i.e. you actually got out of bed to survive and this figure illustrates your survival drives, and no self-actualisation either!).

These models provide food for thought when trying to introduce the new trainee to the practice – all trainers have to do is make them feel happy, stimulated and clever, free and loved – it's that simple!

That's enough preamble – what about some practical points?

THE APPOINTMENT OF GP TRAINEES

Gone are they days when trainers would advertise for, and select, trainees themselves. From April 2000, recruitment to vocational training schemes and general practice placements has been the responsibility of the Directors of Post-graduate General Education.

The aim is to ensure that the recruitment process is open and fairly based on the principles of equal opportunities for all applicants. Part-timers and doctors wishing to return to general practice are positively encouraged. Details of the GP recruitment process can be found at www.gprecruitment.org.uk. Applications are invited twice yearly. The recruitment process is divided into three stages. Trainees submit an online application and if successful will proceed to a written assessment. The final stage involves a face-to-face assessment, which will have three elements:

1 patient simulation exercise
2 written exercise
3 group exercise.

These are discussed in more detail at www.gprecruitment.org.uk. The take-home message is that there are no longer interviews (difficult to standardise and more open to contention), and in order to be successful you must have skills in prioritising, patient communication and working in a group setting.

It should be noted that, due to the 'centralising' of the application process, it is harder for trainees to obtain their 'geographical' choice. Therefore, there will be more trainees having to travel long distances for their placements. This should be kept in mind in relation to their motivation and settling into the practice. Furthermore, the assessment days require huge numbers of assessors, so you will find it will probably be an 'expectation' in your contract that you will be involved to some degree in the selection process.

In summary, the common theme is that trainees are more likely to be choosing you than the other way around. All the more reason to make your practice as attractive as possible to potential trainees. The exact method by which trainees choose their practice can vary between schemes. In some areas trainees are allocated, whereas others may be allowed to visit a number of practices and state their preferences.

WHAT INFORMATION DO TRAINERS PREPARE FOR TRAINEES?

Induction information is an essential part of settling in a new trainee. In the past, this was in written form, and often still is, although increasingly this is based around practice websites. The format may have changed over the years, for example it may now be a section on the practice intranet. Whatever format you use, ensure someone is tasked with reviewing it each year to check it is up to date. An out-of-date set of guidelines will not impress an incoming trainee.

The main issue is to get the balance of information right: too much, and it will never be looked at. Going back to Maslow's hierarchy – think about what the trainee needs to get started and feel more in control. This information will alter over the years – asking your current learner what they have found most useful will be helpful in modifying it for future learners.

This sort of resource is a common tool and should contain a lot of useful information. The following list can be used as a checklist to consider inclusions. It also acts as a reminder of the areas to cover with new trainees even if not formally put in writing:
➤ an index
➤ an introduction to the booklet, stressing where to get help and DON'T PANIC
➤ a brief practice profile (numbers of patients, characteristics of area, major health needs, pattern of service provision, social activities, etc.)
➤ a timetable: this should give details of surgery times, tutorial and half-day commitments

➤ an introduction to the staff (names, job titles, who to ask about what, staff structure, etc.)
➤ an introduction to the clinical staff: doctors, nurses, etc. (names, qualifications, interests, addresses, etc.)
➤ geographical data (maps, street maps, etc.)
➤ a 'need to know list' (see www.radcliffepublishing.com/gptrainershandbook) prioritising what to try and pick up quickly (trainees often feel flooded at the start).
➤ a list of telephone numbers (see www.radcliffepublishing.com/gptrainershandbook)
➤ a list of the potential outside visits
➤ a statement of educational philosophy, i.e. why you train
➤ a statement of the trainee's rights and responsibilities with regard to training
➤ practice leaflet
➤ the initial needs assessment package
➤ the relevant regional documentation
➤ the contract for the trainee
➤ sometimes a job description for the trainee
➤ brief notes on the referral process (i.e. where, who, etc.)
➤ a list of available equipment, i.e. auriscope, ophthalmoscope, tendon hammer, tuning fork, stethoscope, fluoroscein, eye loup, visual acuity charts, peak flow meter, dermatome chart, asthma inhalers for demonstration, weight scales and height measure, tongue depressor, sonicaid, urinalysis sticks, glucometers, speculum, etc.
➤ other available equipment in the surgery, i.e. audiometry, proctoscope, spirometer, sigmoidoscope, arterial doppler, 24-hour BP monitor, pregnancy tests, cautery, cryocautery, curette, autoclave, centrifuge, microscope, resuscitation equipment
➤ a library and IT use advice guide
➤ an introductory timetable and weekly timetable
➤ an introduction to the day-release course
➤ an introduction to MRCGP
➤ an introduction to the use of video
➤ administrative/financial advice
➤ advice on relevant practice policies/procedures, i.e. venepuncture, minor surgery, chaperones, communication within the PHCT, result notification system, visit and telephone contact systems, mail systems and clinical protocols where appropriate
➤ a list of dates to cover regional courses, half-day releases, MRCGP deadlines
➤ other (articles in doctor's bag, etc.).

That is a daunting list – for both trainee and trainer. However, once written it is easy to keep up to date. As long as it treated as a reference manual and not a tome for rote learning, then the feedback from trainees is usually good. A nice addition is a section for the outgoing trainees to add any useful comments for the next incumbent. It can also be helpful to get feedback from previous trainees on what would be helpful to include in an induction pack.

WHAT DO TRAINERS PLAN IN AN INTRODUCTORY COURSE?

The trainee needs a gentle introduction to general practice. Why? For the majority of trainees, they will have come from a hospital-based environment. General practice will come with a much more 'independent' feel.

An induction programme should always be planned in advance, but it will be worth allocating time to review it with the trainee to see if anything can be tailored for their specific learning needs.

Most practices plan a specific one- to two-week induction course for trainees. Most will have similar components which will include:

STRUCTURAL COMPONENTS

Joint surgeries and visits with many partners

This allows the trainee to develop the 'belonging' concept, pick up many of the practical tips and begin to appreciate different consultation styles. This will begin to illustrate that there is no 'one and only' way to consult. I remember being a trainee sat in with various doctors. Each would say at some point 'you are so lucky seeing how the others consult, I would love to do that'. I would sit there feeling slightly guilty that I wasn't sure what I was looking for! One way to help is to prime the trainee with a filter, i.e. attempt to focus there attention without being too directive. This can be pre-written in their diaries or done as a sort of prompt-card (*see* Box 2.1).

BOX 2.1 *Prompt-card example*

Prompt-card for joint surgery with partner A

Every doctor is the best doctor in the world at one thing – but they don't know what it is! Can you find it?
And learn it?
What does partner A do well? How could you learn this?
What does partner A do that surprises you? Why does it surprise you?
Did you ask why s/he did this?

Some of your colleagues may not be as comfortable with having a trainee. Take time to discuss this with them in advance. Let them know what is expected of them as well as of the trainee.

Results from the survey shows that trainers still value joint surgeries and sitting in with the PHCT but that each session should be 'goal orientated'. Some trainers have said that arranging for trainees to sit in again towards the end of the year can also be helpful. At this stage they are looking at consultations in a different way.

Joint surgeries with other PHCT members

For example: practice nurse, health visitor, physiotherapist and district nurse, etc. Again, it is imperative that the trainee considers what they should learn from these sessions. Ideally, we should be aiming to close the loop by following up on the session. Consider whether the PHCT member involved requires any training in teaching techniques. Also consider the specific strengths of each member, e.g. practice nurses teaching travel medicine, sessions with a Macmillan nurse or visiting the local hospice can be invaluable.

Other elements include time spent in the office looking at appointments if taking visit requests. Visiting the local chemist can also be useful.

The concept of home visits will be new to most trainees. Even before they start the unfamiliar skill of consulting in the patient's own home, they have to find there way there! Although we now live in a world of satellite navigation, it can still be helpful to show the trainee local landmarks, common places to visit and any handy little shortcuts. You may consider giving them a list of local places to visit during their induction.

Session with administrator

The actual person to do this may vary but the content needs to cover the essentials of salary, allowances (relocation, telephone, car, etc.), professional details (hopefully already checked, i.e. Medical Defence, GMC certificate) and other administrative detail (phone numbers, addresses, accommodation, on-call details, surgery alarm numbers, relevant keys). Never assume anything. There have been plenty of instances of trainees appearing on day one with expired medical defence, no driving licence, etc. Ensuring that paperwork is correct is beneficial for both parties and allays one of the trainee's biggest stresses – when and how they get paid!

Regional paperwork

Most regions bombard the trainee with booklets on MRCGP and introductory courses. Sometimes it seems weeks before the trainee is allowed to feel it is time to settle into the practice. A warning that many feel like this can help.

Tutorials

The first few tutorials usually cover the 'essentials' – whatever *they* are! In practice, they seem to cover:

➤ prescription forms
➤ essential practice systems
➤ basic computer use
➤ common presentations
➤ contraception
➤ the ill child
➤ the PHCT
➤ sick notes/fit notes
➤ the doctor's bag.*

*This is pretty self-explanatory. Trainees will probably be unfamiliar with what items they should take with them on home visits. It is helpful to show them your own bag and give an idea of what is useful.

Remember to leave time to check any burning issues/queries that may have occurred during the induction process.

PROCESS ELEMENTS

Educational philosophy

In order to foster the learning environment, this is the time to start the role modelling process. It is also the time to introduce motivating processes (fun, competition, belongingness, freedom). In summary, the trainee should have a stimulating, enjoyable, challenging and personally rewarding introduction. Not always easy within a busy practice!

Video

Although the video is no longer assessed as part of the examination, it is still an important tool for teaching consultation skills. The principles of avoiding 'video allergy' still apply:

➤ address any technical difficulties
➤ start early in training
➤ show the trainee a video of yourself consulting.

e-portfolio

MRCGP and its components of assessment are discussed in Chapters 3 and 4. The message is the same as for video. Discuss early so that trainees can get in the habit of using the e-portfolio. You may even want to start discussing the cost of the examinations. These days they really need budgeting for.

SUMMARY

Trainees need an introduction to the practice. This is probably the one area that can be standardised for most trainees. It serves as a secure basis to build on. It allows both the trainee and the trainer time to settle in, time to plan and time to allow the educational process to develop. The concept of role modelling appears to be an essential element of professional education and this period provides the ideal opportunity to show the new trainee a variety of good role models. After all this, perhaps, the trainee and trainer should take the Mad Hatter's advice – sit down and have a cup of tea.

CHAPTER 3

Assessment of learning: how do trainers assess learning needs?

WORKPLACE-BASED ASSESSMENT (WPBA) AND THE MRCGP

Introduction

This section has a particularly circumscribed objective – we aim to identify resources and advice on how to help trainees and trainers deal with the requirements of WPBA and the MRCGP.

There is a vast amount of advice and information available in this area and this section aims to highlight and comment on these resources.

What is WPBA?

Some describe this as the jewel in the crown of the MRCGP – we have one of the first medical assessment processes that involves trainees being assessed doing the job. How much the jewel sparkles depends on the educational process – so we are back to trainers again! (Or Educational and Clinical Supervisors in MRCGP parlance.)

The RCGP definition on WPBA is:

> Workplace-based assessment (WPBA) is defined as the evaluation of a doctor's progress over time in their performance in those areas of professional practice best tested in the workplace. It is a process through which evidence of competence in independent practice is gathered in a structured and systematic framework. Evidence is collected over all three years of training. The evidence is recorded in a web-based portfolio (the e-portfolio) and used to inform six monthly reviews and, at the end of training, to make a holistic, qualitative judgement about the readiness of the GPStR for independent practice.
>
> WPBA is a developmental process. It will therefore provide feedback to the GPStR and drive learning. It will also indicate where a doctor is in difficulty. It is learner led: the GPStR decides which evidence to put forward for review and validation by the trainer.
>
> RCGP

Why WPBA?

Traditional examinations were often based on demonstrating theoretical knowledge and it was inferred that this translated to effective practice – a somewhat

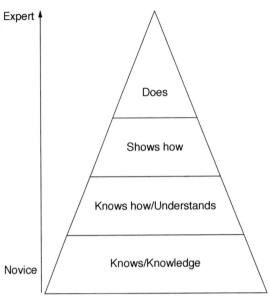

Figure 3.1: Miller's pyramid.

dubious assumption although some might argue this and the apprentice system stood the test of at least 2000 years of medical education! However, current education philosophy and our current curriculum is based on a competency model that is underpinned by a number of educational theories. Miller's Pyramid (*see* Figure 3.1) shows how WPBA attempts to assess as near the apex as possible.

This pyramid can be expanded and more details on this can be seen at: www.gp-training.net/training/educational_theory/adult_learning/miller.htm You could even try the original work: Miller GE. The assessment of clinical skills/competence/performance. *Acad Med.* 1990; 65(9): 63–7.

What are the components of WPBA in GP training?

This section will describe the structural elements of WPBA. There are seven main components of WPBA and these are:

1   multi-source feedback (MSF)
2   patient satisfaction survey (PSQ)
3   consultation observation tool (COT)
4   case-based discussion (CBD)
5   direct observation of procedural skills (DOPS)
6   clinical evaluation exercise (Mini CEX)
7   clinical supervisor's report (CSR).

The Bradford VTS website contains excellent short guides on everything from minimum numbers through to examples of technique for all the various WPBA competence areas. *See* the site at: www.bradfordvts.co.uk/MRCGP/mrcgp.htm

The WPBA components can be mapped onto the RCGP competencies areas as shown in Table 3.1.

Table 3.1 RCGP competence areas

Competence area	MSF	PSQ	COT	CBD	CEX	CSR
Communication and consultation skills	X	X	X		X	X
Practising holistically		X	X	X		X
Data gathering and interpretation	X		X	X	X	X
Making a diagnosis/decision	X		X	X	X	X
Clinical management	X		X	X	X	X
Managing medical complexity				X	X	X
Primary care admin and IT				X		
Working with colleagues	X			X		
Community orientation				X		
Maintaining performance, learning and teaching	X				X	
Maintaining an ethical approach	X			X		
Fitness to practise	X			X		

What is WPBA assessing?

The RCGP comes to the rescue again here (*see* Table 3.2).

Table 3.2

1 **Communication and consultation skills:** this competence is about communication with patients, and the use of recognised consultation techniques.
2 **Practising holistically:** the ability of the doctor to operate in physical, psychological, socioeconomic and cultural dimensions, taking into account feelings as well as thoughts.
3 **Data gathering and interpretation:** the gathering and use of data for clinical judgement, the choice of physical examination and investigations, and their interpretation.
4 **Making a diagnosis/making decisions:** this competence is about a conscious, structured approach to decision-making.
5 **Clinical management:** the recognition and management of common medical conditions in primary care.
6 **Managing medical complexity and promoting health:** aspects of care beyond managing straightforward problems, including the management of co-morbidity, uncertainty, risk and the approach to health rather than just illness.
7 **Primary care administration and IMT:** the appropriate use of primary care administration systems, effective record-keeping and information technology for the benefit of patient care.
8 **Working with colleagues and in teams:** working effectively with other professionals to ensure patient care, including the sharing of information with colleagues.
9 **Community orientation:** the management of the health and social care of the practice population and local community.
10 **Maintaining performance, learning and teaching:** maintaining the performance and effective continuing professional development of oneself and others.

Who does what?

Perhaps a 'Hollywood' analogy might help here.

➤ The trainee is the 'star' – the trainee has to perform and demonstrate the knowledge, skills and attitudes to perform the role.

➤ The trainer or clinical supervisor (CS) (*see* Box 3.1) is the 'director' – the trainer or CS facilitates/directs the star to get the right performance. They make a judgement whether the performance is satisfactory or unsatisfactory and make recommendations for improvement/definition of learning needs/how to achieve new learning objectives. They conduct 'formative' assessments to improve performance.

➤ The educational supervisor (ES) (*see* Box 3.1) is the 'producer' – a film producer is someone who creates the scenes and conditions for making movies – the ES checks that processes are being followed by all the crew, that the production is as planned (the competencies are evidenced appropriately) and that things are running to timetable (progress is satisfactory).

➤ The ARCP Panel are the 'film board': they award the broadcasting certificate (CCT).

BOX 3.1

Clinical supervisor

Clinical supervisors oversee the day-to-day work of the trainee. They are expected to hold formative meetings with their trainee at the beginning, middle and end of their placement. They will be the trainee's initial point of contact in issues relating to the specific post. Clinical supervisors will sign off workplace-based assessments, and write an end-of-placement clinical supervisor's report to be recorded in the trainee's e-portfolio. Trainees and clinical supervisors should at all times be aware of their responsibilities for the safety of patients in their care.

Educational supervisor

Each trainee has a GP educational supervisor who will oversee their progress throughout the entire training programme. Educational supervisors will hold a structured review meeting with the trainee every six months, whatever the length of the practice post. The educational supervisor assesses progress on the basis of workplace-based evidence collected by the trainee and recorded in an e-portfolio. This generates a learning plan and can also be used to identify those trainees in difficulty. These regular reviews do not replace formative meetings with clinical supervisors. The educational supervisor will also conduct appraisals with the trainee.

What resources are there for trainers on the various components of WPBA?

1   The RCGP website: www.rcgp-curriculum.org.uk/nmrgcp/wpba.aspx
2   The Bradford VTS website: www.bradfordvts.co.uk/ED_SUPERVISION/ tipsforTrainees.htm Useful short advice on everything!
3   Deighan M. *The Learning and Teaching Guide*. London: Royal College of General Practitioners; 2007. www.rcgp-curriculum.org.uk/PDF/curr_The_ Learning_and_Teaching_Guide_dec08.pdf
4   Swanwick T and Chana N. Workplace assessment for licensing in general practice. Discussion Paper. *British Journal of General Practice*. June 2005: 461–7.
5   Chana N, Gardiner P, Rughani A and Williams N. *Talking the Talk: using case-based discussion in medical assessments*. London: Royal College of General Practitioners; 2007. This DVD and accompanying workbook on case-based discussion is on sale from the RCGP Bookshop.
6   Planning and Conducting the CbD Interview: available on the RCGP MRCGP website at: www.rcgp.org.uk/docs/MRCGP_How%20to%20 plan%20and%20conduct%20the%20CBD%20interview.doc This single sheet describes the CbD process.
7   CbD Structured Question Guidance: available on the RCGP MRCGP website at: www.rcgp.org.uk/docs/MRCGP_CBD%20Structured%20 Question%20Guidance.do This is a single sheet of advice usefully highlighting facilitation questions – very useful to give to other clinicians acting as educational supervisors for a CbD session.
8   COT: Detailed Guide to the Performance Criteria. Available on the RCGP MRCGP website at: www.rcgp.org.uk/docs/MRCGP_COT_Guide_to_ Performance_Criteria.doc This sheet gives useful descriptors for all of the performance criteria.
9   MRCGP DVD: *The COT. A Guide to the Consultation Observation Tool*. Available from the RCGP bookshop and from the Wessex faculty office. £25, with discounts for RCGP members and associates. Discounts for bulk orders from the Wessex faculty office.
10 The multi-source feedback questionnaire is available as a Word document on the RCGP MRCGP website at: www.rcgp.org.uk/docs/MRCGP_msf%20 form%20from%20e-portfolio.doc
11 A copy of the PSQ can be downloaded from the RCGP MRCGP website at: www.rcgp.org.uk/Docs/MRCGP_all%20six%20assessment%20forms.doc

What is required and when?

See Table 3.3.

Table 3.3

MSF	Multi-source feedback	Two in ST1 (five clinical) and two in ST3 (five clinical and five non-clinical)
Mini CEX	Mini clinical evaluation exercise	Hospital-based equivalent to COT
DOPS	Direct observation of procedural skills	Nine mandatory procedures – witnessed and accredited
CbD	Case-based discussions	Six in ST1, six in ST2, 12 in ST3
COT	Consultation observation tool	General practice tool for live observation or using video
CSR	Clinical supervisor's report	After every hospital and GP attachment
PSQ	Patient satisfaction questionnaire	One in every GP attachment –at least 40 patients

What are the core skills trainers use in WPBA?

These can be summarised as:
➤ organisational
➤ observational
➤ analytical
➤ validation
➤ assessment
➤ standard setting
➤ feedback
➤ teaching
➤ motivational
➤ managerial
➤ role modelling.

We will look at tools trainers use in these areas across many chapters, but will look at a few specific ones here that seem to underpin the success of this process.

Reflection

The process of reflection underpins teaching the learner and educator alike. Gibbs' reflective cycle (*see* Figure 3.2 and http://distributedresearch.net/wiki/index.php/Gibbs_reflective_Cycle) helps to encourage a wider analysis of an event and can be combined with the logical levels of neurolinguistic planning. The latter can be written out as floor tiles with the trainee hopping from one to the other as they look at a particular chosen event. The trainer then facilitates discussion, using each level to help the trainees develop reflective insights at each level (*see* Table 3.4).

The following questions can be a helpful adjunct:
Q1   Where are you? (scene setting)
Q2   What is the problem? Area for change? (clarifying goal)
Q3   How do you feel about this? (feelings)

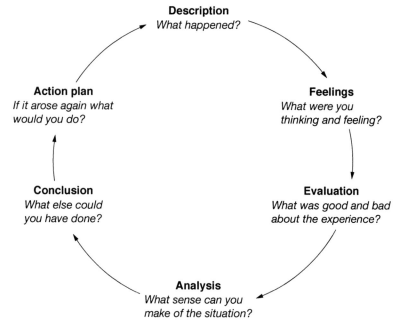

Figure 3.2: Gibbs' reflective cycle (from *Learning by Doing: a guide to teaching and learning methods*; 1988).

Table 3.4

Spirituality	How does this fit into my view of the wider world?
Identity	Who am I here? How do I perceive myself? How do I want to be perceived?
Values	What do I really value in this situation? Are my core values being challenged?
Beliefs	What do I believe? Is it justifiable? Is it consistent with the evidence?
Capability	What skills does this situation need? Have I got them? How can access/develop them?
Behaviour	How am I behaving here? Why? Is it helpful?
Environment	Is the environment helping or hindering? What external factors are having an impact?

Q4   What are you thinking about this? (thoughts)
Q5   What do these thoughts mean? (interpretation)
Q6   Why do you believe they mean this? (values)
Q7   Who are you? (personal comfort/role)
Q8   Are you comfortable with your beliefs (beliefs)
Q9   Is change still necessary? (check problem still real)
Q10 Name a specific change you can make? (identify change)

Even Kipling's 'Six serving men' can be useful in a quick 'microteaching' environment:

I keep six honest serving-men
(They taught me all I knew);
Their names are What and Why and When
And How and Where and Who.

The basic cycle of cognitive behavioural theory is another useful model to help trainees with the added advantage of having a direct link to clinical care. Figure 3.3 shows the basic cognitive behavioural theory cycle – *see* Chapter 6 for a description of its use in practice.

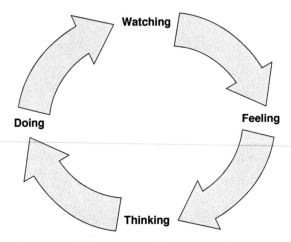

Figure 3.3: Kolb's experiential learning cycle, version 1.

This section would be incomplete without some thoughts on learning cycles. Perhaps the two most commonly mentioned names here are Schon and Kolb. Schon wrote extensively about reflection and some of his concepts are usefully remembered (*see* Schon D. *Educating the Reflective Practitioner: towards a new design for teaching and learning in the Professions.* Oxford: Jossey Bass; 1987).

➤ **Tacit knowledge** – this is the knowledge we have derived from experience and it emerges in context. Some have described it as 'situational certainty' and it develops into 'knowing in action', i.e. the competent performance. It is, however, not open to easy analysis – a bit like the unconsciously competent practitioner – and encourages the learner and educator to look for these competencies.

➤ **Reflection in action** – this develops when the learner becomes aware that the performance is in some way unexpected. This situation opens the opportunity for new learning but may not always be captured.

➤ **Reflection on action** – this is hopefully where the opportunity for learning is captured with the concept of learning in action, widening the potential learning.

Kolb's Experiential Learning Cycle (*see* Figure 3.3) is seen in many guises but perhaps is most useful in its simplest form.

As soon as the educationalists get at it, things get more complicated – and this is just the start – if you want to read more try: www.businessballs.com/kolblearningstyles.htm (*see* Figure 3.4).

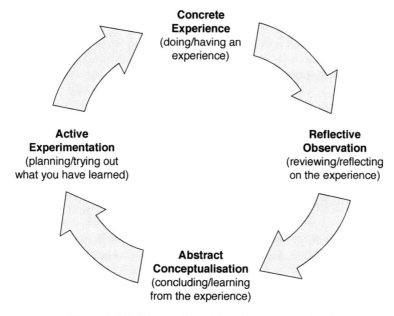

Figure 3.4 Kolb's experiential learning cycle, version 2.

These models can help trainers develop reflective habits in trainees (*see* Chapter 6).

We will look at learning style tools in a later chapter but perhaps the most commonly mentioned is the *Learning Style Inventory* by Peter Honey at: www.peterhoney.com/content/LearningStylesQuestionnaire.html This inventory can help identify how well learners will adapt to a more intense reflective process.

The literature on learning styles has expanded enormously and a good overview site can be found at: www.learning-styles-online.com/

Feedback

> We must remember to talk about goodness everyday (Socrates)

Feedback underpins all learning – deceptively easy if it is in a positive vein but most trainers find this difficult outside this area. This is probably related to our past humiliations at the hands of previous teachers and our enduring fear of failure. It is very difficult to give feedback if you still harbour these feelings. Successful feedback is given in an atmosphere where it is accepted as an essential and positive ingredient of the learning process. So basically you must give *and receive* it regularly, openly, honestly, positively *and* negatively. Box 3.2 shows the principles that should be used.

BOX 3.2 *Principles for feedback*

➤ Owned (i.e. use of 'I' not 'we'), NOT implied.
➤ Planned, NOT impulsive.
➤ Honest, NOT collusive.
➤ Valid, NOT irrelevant (i.e. apply to a shared agenda).
➤ Concerned, NOT destructive.
➤ Specific, NOT vague.
➤ Behaviour, NOT the person.
➤ Observation, NOT inference.
➤ Sooner, NOT later.
➤ Descriptive, NOT judgemental.
➤ Sharing ideas, NOT giving advice.
➤ Exploring alternatives, NOT providing answers.
➤ Good, NOT only bad (i.e. balanced and reinforcing good learning).

The trainer needs courage, understanding, self-respect and skills as well as a respect for the trainee. The focus should be on behaviour that is amenable to change and the feedback should be prescribed in a manner analogous to drug prescribing, i.e.:
➤ correctly timed
➤ in the right dose (not too little or too much)
➤ with clarity and accuracy
➤ when the correct indication exists, i.e. the feedback will work
➤ with the trainee's concordance
➤ with explicit conditions for follow-up
➤ for the trainee's benefit (not the trainer's!).

The 'feedback sandwich' is a practical reminder of the need to provide feedback with protection, particularly if you have an under-confident trainee. This simply implies that you wrap the constructive criticism in two layers of positive comment. A lot of feedback is simple and straightforward, but the trainer needs to be sensitive to the feelings it can produce in the trainee before the feedback session is closed.

The Standing Committee of Postgraduate Medical Education (SCOPME) suggests a nine-point plan:

1 listen to the trainee
2 reflect back points for clarification
3 give support
4 counsel
5 treat information in confidence
6 inform without censure
7 judge constructively
8 identify educational needs
9 negotiate and construct an achievable learning plan.

If this is an obvious problem for a trainee the following techniques can be tried:
➤ a tutorial where trainer/trainee describe the best/worst feedback they have ever had
➤ a tutorial where the trainer/trainee role play a feedback scenario.

Trainers should always remember that a quick 'That's right! Well done' reinforces learning very effectively. Similarly, negative feedback should be given without unnecessary repetition.

Specific teaching tools
Questions and answers

> As long as the answer is right, who cares if the question is wrong? (Jung)

Any parent will testify to the truth that asking questions is easier than answering them!

One of the key skills in developing a trainee's self-directed learning approach is the use of appropriate questions. In the training environment questions are not answered – they are questioned! Four types of question can be used.
1 Direct questions
   – a question seeking an answer or sequence of answers.
2 Probing questions
   – with cues
   – with elaboration
   – with explanation
   – to provoke knowledge seeking
   – to involve others (perhaps in a group).
3 High order questions: i.e. broadening the area, seeking justifications.
   (These are questions that provoke thought, bring out principles or require problem solving skills.)
4 Divergent questions: i.e. hypotheses or alternatives seeking.

Questions that open awareness often have no 'right' answer and encourage creative thinking.

Trainees can find these approaches frustrating if they are new to this kind of teaching. It can help if trainers make the reasons for this style explicit. It can be very rewarding when trainees produce their own solutions with a smile and the trainer hadn't even thought of one!

Teaching clinical examination and procedures (see DOPS)

The following sequence has been suggested as a guide to use when teaching clinical skills in the clinical setting.

➤ Set the environment.
➤ Introduce and inform everyone.
➤ Work out and describe the sequence of actions that are required.
➤ Demonstrate the process as you would normally perform it.
➤ Use imagery/models to illustrate the process.
➤ Check the trainee understanding of the process.
➤ The trainee performs the process under supervision.
➤ Focus sensory awareness on key elements (i.e. close eyes).
➤ Build confidence with feedback and practice.
➤ Use linkage:
   – facts to feelings
   – visual to other sensory inputs
   – clinical history to examination findings.
➤ Increase responsibility (trainee does it alone).
➤ Check on progress at agreed time interval.

Although the points seem obvious, it does challenge the trainer to define the skills required and to develop a bank of teaching strategies and linkage techniques for this process. This has become more critical as the DOPS process defines a number of essential procedures (and optional others). It can be an interesting exercise to take these procedures and work through these stages. Most trainers will find a number of aspects they had assumed (i.e. they were unconscious competence) that the trainee was skilled in. These assumptions may, or may not, be correct and are usefully highlighted.

Teaching GP clinical strategies

Many trainees have developed a hospital-based approach to diagnosis and examination. Most rapidly learn to adapt this approach. The Family Medicine Department in UBC Vancouver raises this process to a conscious level by working through common presentations using a number of set questions. The form used is reproduced in the appendix to this chapter and at www.radcliffe publishing.com/gptrainershandbook. The process can be useful in two areas.

First, to help the trainee who is having difficulty adapting to the primary care environment, and secondly to look at a particular presentation that a trainee may be struggling with. Trainers need to consider the potential problem of giving the message that there is always a single set of 'right' questions for a particular presentation but, with this proviso, the method could be helpful.

The micro-lesson 'CATCH-ing' the learning opportunity

This phrase was coined by one trainer and coincides with a concept developed from Irby by Dr Bob Woollard in the UBC Vancouver Family Medicine Department. Much of our one-to-one teaching involves short interactions with the trainee between consultations or actually with patients present. Six 'micro-skills' for the teacher can be developed to act as a guide to maximise the learning potential in this situation.

Commitment:	The trainer should ask the learner for a commitment to the problem (i.e. diagnosis, reason for attendance, problem definition). This involves clarification of the learner's knowledge base in relation to presentation and management issues.
Analysis:	The trainer should now ask for a demonstration of the reasoning behind the assessment. This allows the learner's problem-solving skills to be demonstrated.
Teaching:	The trainer can now assess the need for new knowledge and help with problem solving. This is the time to bring out the principles or concepts that apply in the situation, i.e. some teaching.
Compliments:	The power of positive feedback can never be underestimated. The trainer should say specifically what was done well and what effect this has had. Opportunities for reinforcement of good practice should never be missed.
Howlers:	Obvious mistakes, omissions and misunderstandings should highlight learning needs and these should be appropriately fed back.

Some trainers add a caveat here – 'CATCH-1' – the original model potentially ends on a negative note and adding 'one' more point can change this – perhaps identifying a particular learning need or reinforcing a particularly good point.

Further chapters will offer some tools to help trainers analyse, motivate, validate and model their learners.

The Chicago model

This is another 'micro-teaching' model described in Wall D, Chambers R and Mohanna K. *Teaching Made Easy: A Manual for Healthcare Professionals.* Oxford: Radcliffe Medical Press; 2004.

1   Review aims and objectives at the start: 'Begin at the beginning.'
2   Give interim feedback of a positive nature 'Set a positive tone.'
3   Ask for learner self-appraisal: 'Ask before telling.'
4   Give feedback on behaviours: 'Behaviour not person.'
5   Give specific examples: 'Evidence not opinion.'
6   Suggest strategies to improve learning: 'Build up not knock down.'

The six-step model
This is a rather neat aide-memoire for micro-teaching:
1   problem presented
2   problem discussed
3   problem agreed
4   solution proposed
5   solution discussed
6   solution agreed.

A reflective equation

$$WD_{LB} + LU_{BB} = Learning$$

This translates to Write Down in Little Book + Look Up in Big Book. Perhaps in the modern era it should be WDLB + LUKS – look up in knowledge source?

PUNs/DENs
This is now quite a well-known concept: Patient Unmet Needs become Doctor's Educational Needs. However, as a group we are still not good at capturing the learning potential of our consultations and using these ideas can increase the potential for learning.

THE APPLIED KNOWLEDGE TEST (AKT)

This is a three-hour online multiple choice question (MCQ) test with 200 questions covering the knowledge base that underpins UK general practice, with sittings three times a year in DVLA testing centres.

What are the areas covered by the AKT?
The AKT tests topics that are common and/or important in three main categories:
1 core clinical medicine and its application to problem solving in a general practice context **80%**
2 critical appraisal and evidence-based clinical practice **10%**
3 health administration, informatics and the organisational structures that support UK general practice. **10%**

Key messages: the exam is mostly about *applied* knowledge in a *clinical* context, not knowledge per se. The performance of examinees in critical appraisal is generally very poor. A little knowledge in this area can therefore earn valuable marks.

RCGP

Trainers have had the following thoughts on how to help trainees with the AKT.

1 Tell them to look at:
   - guidelines (www.eguidelines.co.uk)
   - SIGN
   - NICE documents
   - BNF
   - DVLA guidance
   - DWP guidance (fit notes, etc. – *see* 'Forms you should know' in Chapter 4)
   - immunisation guidance ('The Green Book')
   - statistics (statistical and evidence-based medicine resources include books (Greenhalgh T. *How to Read a Paper.* Chichester: Wiley Blackwell BMJ Books; 2010; Harris M. *Medical Statistics Made Easy.* London: Informa Healthcare; 2003; Crombie I. *The Pocket Guide to Critical Appraisal.* London: BMJ Publications; 2006); or try http://dorakmt. tripod.com/mtd/glosstat.html for definitions).
   - some specific books (Kumar P and Clarke M. *Clinical Medicine.* 6th ed. London: Elselvier; 2010; *Oxford Handbook of General Practice.* Oxford: Oxford University Press; 2006), particularly for practice management issues, were mentioned.
2 Advise them to join a study group.
3 Tell them to read the condensed statements in the RCGP curriculum guide to avoid any 'black holes'.
4 Set a target date for the AKT.
5 Get some practice (*see* the RCGP website and www.passmedicine.com, www.oneexamination.com, www.pastest.co.uk).
6 Have a tutorial on technique – often the questions have some easily excludable options – often leaving two infuriatingly difficult to decide between! Looking *very carefully* at the question again can help (examiners sweat blood over these questions and often a cue is hidden in the wording). If undecided, annotate the question and plough on (allowing for a bit of subconscious reasoning to occur).
7 Practice doing the questions at a suitable rate – enough to allow 15–20 minutes at the end to review annotated ones.
8 Buy some attempts at the online RCGP AKT and do some them together as a tutorial.

9   Try writing some AKT-type questions together.
10   The bottom-line advice is to consider what you personally would do in
     the clinical situation – usually this is a good pointer in the right direction.

The following resources may be helpful in these areas.

Statistical terms

> The best way to understand a term is to explain it to someone else (Anon)

This list has been used as a pairs exercise to raise awareness of the terms. The
trainer and trainee or trainee pairs work down the list in Table 3.5 taking
explaining alternate terms to each other. The definitions are available in the
books/websites mentioned above.

Table 3.5

RANDOMISED	BIAS	PROSPECTIVE	RETROSPECTIVE	DOUBLE BLIND
DROPOUTS	POWER	SPECIFICITY	SENSITIVITY	POSITIVE PREDICTIVE VALUE
VALIDITY	RELIABILITY	SIGNIFICANCE	OUTCOME	ENDPOINT
CONFIDENCE INTERVAL	RECRUITMENT	BLIND	GENERALISABILITY	OBSERVATIONAL
COHORT	LONGITUDINAL	CROSS SECTIONAL	INTERVENTIONAL	CASE-CONTROL
ABSOLUTE RISK REDUCTION (ARR)		RELATIVE RISK (RR) REDUCTION		STANDARD DEVIATION
CHI-SQUARED TEST	MODE	CORRELATION COEFFICIENT	MEAN	P-VALUE
NUMBER NEEDED TO TREAT (NNT)				

Critical appraisal

The shortened schema in Box 3.3 can be used to look at a paper in a tutorial.

BOX 3.3

ENVIRONMENT   Who did the study? Why? Where? Is it relevant to
                 ordinary general practice?
OBJECTIVES   Are they stated? If not can you deduce them?
DESIGN   What is it?
          case report   *prospective*
          case series   *retrospective*

---

cross sectional	*intervention/non-intervention*
longitudinal	*experimental*
case control	*controlled trial*
cohort	

Is it relevant to the study objective stated?

Could you reproduce it from the details given?

SAMPLE CHARACTERISTICS

Representative?

What was the sampling method? Was bias introduced? (selection/observer/recall)

Sample size? Are there statistics to show it is large enough?

Entry criteria

Exclusions

Non-respondents

CONTROL GROUP CHARACTERISTICS

How were controls defined?

What was their source?

How were they matched/randomised?

What is the effect of comparable factors?

QUALITY OF MEASUREMENTS/OUTCOMES

Test characteristics, i.e. validity/sensitivity/specificity/reproducibility/reliability

Blindness?

Quality control, i.e. calibration exercises/observer repeatability tests

Outcome measures, i.e. defined/valid

COMPLETENESS

Dropouts/deaths

Missing data

Response rates?

RESULTS

Are they well laid out?

What about the statistics?

DISTORTING INFLUENCES

Contamination, i.e. cases in control group, etc.

Confounding variables

Time effects

Analysis distortions

Sponsorship?

CONCLUSIONS

Are they justified?

Reference: Foulkes F and Fulton P. Critical appraisal of published literature. *BMJ.* 1991; **2**: 121–5.

READER

This is a critical appraisal tool described in MacAuley D. READER: An acronym to aid critical reading in general practice. *Br Gen Pract.* 1994; **44**: 83–5. It can be a simple aide-memoir when reading a publication.

R	Relevance	* To the GP
		* To your own circumstance/patient
		* General awareness
E	Education	* Would it change your behaviour?
		* Would it challenge your beliefs?
A	Applicability	* Does it seem applicable in your practice?
		* Are the results generalisable?
D	Discrimination	* What is the quality of the study?
		* What sort of study is it?
		* What about – sample size?
		– bias?
		– selection?
		– controls?
		– study design?
		– statistics?
		– results?
		– conclusions?
E	Evaluation	* Reflect on its overall impact/value
R	Reaction	* What are you now going to do?

THE CLINICAL SKILLS ASSESSMENT (CSA)

This is where trainees demonstrate the integration of their competencies in the 'Tower of Terror' in Croydon.

The CSA

The Clinical Skills Assessment (CSA) is an essential component of the MRCGP, and is 'an assessment of a doctor's ability to integrate and apply clinical, professional, communication and practical skills appropriate for general practice'.

GPStRs will be eligible to take the CSA when they are in ST3 (the third and final year of their GP specialty training).

Trainees see 13 cases at *exactly* 10-minute intervals and are assessed in three areas with one of four possible grades:

➤ clear pass
➤ marginal pass

➤ marginal fail
➤ clear fail.

The three areas are:
A   data gathering, technical and assessment skills
B   clinical management skills
C   interpersonal skills.

These map onto various areas of the curriculum as shown below:

> The CSA tests mainly from the following areas of the curriculum:
>
> **Primary care management** – recognition and management of common medical conditions in primary care. **B**
> **Problem solving skills** – gathering and using data for clinical judgement, choice of examination, investigations and their interpretation. Demonstration of a structured and flexible approach to decision-making. **A**
> **Comprehensive approach** – demonstration of proficiency in the management of co-morbidity and risk. **B**
> **Person-centred care** – communication with patient and the use of recognised consultation techniques to promote a shared approach to managing problems. **C**
> **Attitudinal aspects** – practising ethically with respect for equality and diversity, with accepted professional codes of conduct. **C**
> The CSA will also test:
> **Clinical practical skills** – demonstrating proficiency in performing physical examinations and using diagnostic/therapeutic instruments.
>
> RCGP

What advice do trainers offer to help facilitate this process?

This is a high-pressure, closely observed, high-stakes performance examination – many trainees have only just started managing 10-minute appointments (and many established GPs now book 15-minute appointments as standard) and accept over-running and against this background this is a challenging assessment. Perhaps the first task is to reassure that trainees practising 'good enough' consultations will pass! With that in mind, the following pointers were offered.
➤ Preparing trainees: make sure they understand what this exam is assessing. Use CbD and COT tools to address the specific areas mentioned above. Do some joint surgeries with the same approach. Many trainees will plan to sit this in February leaving time for a re-sit in April/May. Make sure they know the format and can manage 10-minute appointments. Make sure they are prepared for a sudden end to consultations (a 10-minute 'shutter' operates in the exam) and are not too fazed by this.

➤ Each case will have a particular 'focus', i.e. the diagnosis may be easy but it is sharing the management plan that is the issue, the presentation may be physical but depression is the issue. Consider tutorials covering:
  - hidden agendas
  - covert depression
  - 'difficult patients', i.e. angry, not wanting the accepted treatment, having a well-entrenched, unusual health belief, requesting investigation/treatment/referral that is outside 'normal practice', complaining patients, patients who know more than you about something or ask about an area you know little about, asking for certification (watch out for other agenda here)
  - giving concise explanations.
➤ Explore the pass/fail boundary with trainees:

Marginal Pass

The candidate demonstrates an adequate level of competence, displaying a clinical approach that may not be fluent but is justifiable and technically proficient. The candidate shows sensitivity and tried to involve the patient

Marginal Fail

The candidate fails to demonstrate adequate competence, with a clinical approach that is at times unsystematic or inconsistent with accepted practice. Technical proficiency may be of concern. The patient is treated with sensitivity and respect, but the doctor does not sufficiently facilitate or respond to the patient's contribution

RCGP

➤ Courses: 'Practice makes perfect' and these courses can help calm nerves too! The RCGP course has the advantage of actually using the same premises as the exam. Kay Bridgeman's course was commented on very positively but most VTSs run courses too.
➤ Coaching: cover consultations on common conditions, write some cases together – examples can be found in Thakkar R, Havelock P and Barnes A. *MRCGP Practice Cases: clinical skills assessment.* Knutsford: Pastest; 2008. Do a tutorial using role play together using these.
➤ The four most common problem areas (in 2010) are shown in Table 3.6.

Essentially, these comments relate to three areas:
1 Clinical practice – not being aware of current best practice – identifies a need to scope for black holes (use the curriculum statements, other curriculum tools), a need to look at the trainee's knowledge base (practise AKTs, relevant resources mentioned above) and a need to keep seeing patients with 'WHY' in your mind at all times – Why am I doing this?

Table 3.6

Problem area	Advice
Does not develop a management plan (including prescribing and referral) that is appropriate and in line with current best practice of make adequate arrangements for follow up and safety netting.	Practice giving a precise summary of the management plan – make sure the patient understands and agrees (see the points below).
Does not identify patient's health agenda, health beliefs and preferences: does not make use of verbal and non-verbal cues.	Make sure you 'ICE' the patient! Do a tutorial using Helman's Model, write out a series of questions covering these points together as a tutorial, exploring the subtleties of asking about these issue and practice using them.
	Make verbal and non-verbal cues more explicit by identifying them – in joint surgeries, role play and video – explore techniques for responding to these. Identify possible responses and practice them.
Does not develop a shared management plan or clarify the roles of patient and doctor.	Use COT and CbD to look at how this is achieved – are management options explored? To what degree is the patient's agenda explored, considered and used? Look at ways of doing these? Explore why it is not being done?
Does not recognise the challenge (i.e. the patient's main problem, ethical issue, etc.).	Highlight cues that this may be happening, i.e. finishing quickly, feeling awkward, verbal and non-verbal cues – identify techniques for 'starting again' – practice them.

2 Patient-centred practice: trainees still arrive in practice with a 'Hospital-based' approach and often need re-focusing – do a tutorial on this area looking at trainer videos and highlight this behaviour. Explore what competencies address these issues and what skills are needed? Identify strategies to cover this and how to review progress.

3 Make sure 'acting with an actor' is not a problem!

A trainers' meeting recently heard the following pieces of information.

➤ Trainees rarely pass if they have seen fewer than 100 patients in the practice (and they shouldn't pass either!).

➤ The exam rewards 'fluency', i.e. trainees who do well have developed their

own style (behaviours, phrases, etc.) and come across as more natural consulters.
➤ Make sure trainees have a '10-minute awareness', i.e. they can do a 'beginning, middle and end' consultation in that time.
➤ Encourage them to familiarise themselves with the COT criteria.
➤ Try to de-threaten the exam – as one examiner puts it: 'this is the safest surgery you'll ever do!'

Since September 2010 there have been 13 marked cases and the pass mark is determined on the day to even out disparities caused by case mix. Trainers in some areas will be asked what experience/teaching trainees have had if they fail the CSA.

WHAT DOES THE ARCP PANEL THINK ABOUT THE E-PORTFOLIO?

Boxes 3.4 and 3.5 offer some thoughts for trainers and trainees – they are reproduced by the kind permission of Matt Smith of the Pennine VTS.

BOX 3.4 *What the ARCP panel thinks about e-portfolio contents (2010)*

(This summary of RCGP external assessors findings was a poster presentation by I Edwards *et al.* and was based on a review of a 10% sample of e portfolios.)
Trainee log entries
Unacceptable
➤ Descriptive list of learning events.
➤ No reflection of learning or professional development.
➤ Limited range of evidence presented.
➤ Poorly populated learning.
➤ Entries scant and descriptive.

Acceptable
➤ Uses a limited range of evidence-gathering tools.
➤ Some reflection on learning and personal development.
➤ Some contextual application of knowledge and evidence but not well developed.
➤ Some reflection on feedback.

Excellent (in addition to acceptable)
➤ Extensive range of log entries using a wide range of discriminating tools as evidence of competence.
➤ Uses feedback to critically assess developmental needs.

➤ Critical reflection of significant events, e.g. develops a PDP in response to reflection on complaints.
➤ Contextual application and critical appraisal of evidence to justify decisions and development.

Clinical supervisor comments
Unacceptable
➤ Tick box completed inaccurately.
➤ Judgements not referenced to portfolio.
➤ Where judgements can be evaluated, they do not appear to be justifiable.
➤ No comment is made on the current state and progression of competence.
➤ Little or no analysis of trainee strengths and weaknesses.
➤ No suggestions for improvement.
➤ No PDP formulated and agreed with trainee.

Acceptable
➤ Judgements are justifiable and referenced to evidence.
➤ The current state and progress are made clear.
➤ Trainee's strength and weaknesses are identified and described.
➤ Recommendations for further development are evidenced and addresses the needs identified.

Excellent (in addition to acceptable)
➤ Comments are a more sophisticated in-depth analysis of trainee strengths and areas for development.
➤ Efforts made to triangulate evidence with comments based on more than one source.
➤ Critically evaluates evidence to define recommendations for further development.
➤ Supervisor comments on the quality and range of evidence set in order to improve trainee insight into the data.

Education supervisor
Unacceptable
➤ The basis for judgements is not clear and not referenced to the evidence.
➤ Where judgements can be evaluated they do not appear justifiable.
➤ No comment is made on the current state and progress of competence.

➤ Suggestions for trainee development inadequate in number and quality.

Acceptable
➤ Judgements generally referenced to available evidence.
➤ Judgements appear to be justifiable.
➤ Current state of progress of competence is made clear.
➤ Suggestions for trainee are routinely made and appear appropriate.

Excellent (in addition to acceptable)
➤ Judgements show sophisticated synthesising of evidence from a number of sources.
➤ Suggestions for trainee development clarify learning outcomes to be achieved.
➤ Comments on the quality and range of evidence set in order to improve trainee insight into data.

BOX 3.5 *Reflections of an ARCP panel member June 2009*

With our round of ARCP panels just completed, we identified a number of themes which emerged from the discussions at panel this year. One consistent comment from both panels was just how GPST engagement with the e-portfolio and WPBA has improved in the last 12 months. Another recurring comment was just how much the detailed structured educational supervisors' report facilitated panel assessment and discussion.

So here are some of the key learning points and suggestions

1. In every case issues warranting deanery 'face-to-face ARCP panel' referral had been identified at educational supervision, emphasising the importance of GPSTs implementing the recommendations of their educational supervisors.

    In order to minimise the number of GPSTs requiring referral for 'face-to-face' deanery panel review we are suggesting trainers and GPSTs, following the formative educational supervision in March, run through the download from the MRCGP section of the website: www.pennine-gp-training.co.uk/An-Assessment-sheet-for-ARCP--for-Trainers---GPSTs.doc *(a useful tool to employ after the supplementary formative Educational Supervision meeting in March, as it ensures that there is enough time for remedial action prior to the local ARCP panels in June).*

2. A few GPSTs in ST2 who only started their first GP placement in April (prior to the June ARCP panel) have had their 'satisfactory progress' panel outcome held (not signed off by the panel chair) due to a lack of a PSQ. **This emphasises the importance for ST2s starting their first GP placement in April to commence their PSQ in second month of their post, as all 40 responses need to be uploaded by the end of May.**

3. It was also reassuring to *see* that GPSTs and Trainers had heeded the learning points identified from the November round of ARCP panels. I have copied them across from the News section of the website . . .

ARCP Panel Review – Reflections of a panel member from the last round of panels in November 2008

Some of the important recurring questions by panel members were:
➤ Have they logged enough good quality entries (2 entries per week in hospital posts and 3 per week in general practice, as a rough guide)?
➤ Are they of significant breadth and depth (multiple entries in ALL of the domains, e.g. SEA, audit/project, clinical encounters, etc.)?
➤ Have they been mapped to the curriculum (on average 2 or more per log entry) and is the mapping valid?
➤ Is there good curriculum coverage?
➤ Have they completed the minimum numbers of workplace-based assessments (CBDs, COTS, etc.)?
➤ Enough DOPs (DOPs on manikins in isolation don't count!) and OOH sessions?
➤ Are they using their PDP?
➤ What does the ES report say (clear statements by the ES are very helpful)?
➤ What does the CSR reveal (especially if they were from a GP trainer)?
➤ What do the MSFs say about the trainee?
➤ What does the PSQ reveal about their practice (NB MSF was found to be a more important discriminator)?

It is important to reaffirm that the minimum number of e-portfolio entries or WPBAs (COTs, CBDs, etc.) is the minimum and we expect more!

4. We found that trainers and clinical supervisors who entered a simple description of the clinical scenario in the comment section of their CBDs, COTs, etc. helped us interpret the competencies demonstrated.

Overall assessment
Feedback and recommendations for further development
Agreed action
Time taken for discussion (in minutes)
Time taken for feedback (in minutes)

5. As mentioned previously, the detailed structured educational supervisor's report facilitated panel assessment and discussion significantly, especially as ARCP panel members have a restricted e-portfolio view of log entries and no view of the PDP! We have changed the summative educational supervisor's report form to ensure that the information copied across to the e-portfolio covers these key areas. This can be found in the Tools for Educational Supervisors part of the website at: www.pennine-gp-training.co.uk/ Ed-Sup-RCGP-Form.doc

6. Detailed CSR reports by the trainers greatly facilitated educational supervisors completion of the progression of competency which in turn was helpful to panel members.

7. Screening of the e-portfolios by educational supervisors and the panel chair a few weeks prior to panel which generated a few succinct e-mails to GPSTs ensured that the numbers of GPSTs failing panel review due to too few CBDs, COTs, etc. was avoided.

SUMMARY

The RCGP curriculum is a vast achievement and, at first sight, a daunting prospect for trainer and trainee alike. There are a number of resources designed to inform, direct and educate and this chapter has attempted to signpost many of these in an attempt to make the process easier and perhaps even fun!

Our current generation of trainees are purportedly 'generation Y' and, just like our profession is changing, so perhaps are preferred learning environments. Generation Y may learn best when (in rank order):
➤ learning is fun
➤ through mentoring and coaching
➤ with multisensory input
➤ with peers
➤ in social or informal settings.

Interestingly, the same survey (from Talentsmoothie) put computer-based learning below all of the above. Our challenge as trainers is to take all these ingredients and mix them well.

Appendix 1

GP CLINICAL STRATEGIES FORM

This form is a series of questions to work through. The aim is to investigate the techniques that GPs use to manage presentations particularly in relation to the time restraints at work in primary care.

➤ What is the problem/presentation?
➤ What is the worst case scenario?
➤ What are the essential questions?
➤ What are the 'red flags'?
➤ What investigations are indicated?
➤ What aspects of the patient's agenda might be relevant?
➤ Are there any health education aspects of relevance?
➤ Does the trainer know of any 'pearls of wisdom' on this subject?

Useful presentations to consider include (try listing these with the trainee):
➤ TATT
➤ URTIs
➤ rashes
➤ joint pains
➤ headaches
➤ depression
➤ sick note requests
➤ sleep problems
➤ chest pains
➤ SOB.

THE 19-POINT GUIDE TO EDUCATIONAL SUPERVISION

(This guide is based on a presentation by David Palmer, VTS Course Organiser Stafford.)

1 **Preparation**: Log in – check 'educator notes' – check posts – is the clinical supervisor's report (CSR) there ? – is it attached to the right post? Are there two CSRs for the year? (ideally one for every post).

2 Look at the learning log – list all entries, check the date of the last entry. Are working hours documented? Are there any audits/significant event reviews?

3 Check that the learning log links to professional competencies – *justifiably* – may need to prune these. What is the strength of the evidence offered? Look at enough to ensure you feel the trainees approach is satisfactory, i.e. they are demonstrating competence.

4 If ST3 consider advising on how to target evidence at rare competencies – look for 'missed' opportunities (i.e. genetics – saw a Ca breast patient with a strong FH, or maintaining professionalism – presented a significant event review in VTS small group work. Could they use the ESR as a learning event?, etc.).

5 Look at the WPBA – are they good enough? Watch out for the green/red colouring – cannot always rely on green meaning enough are being done at that stage.

6 Look at COTs, CbDs, DOPS, MSFs . . . right numbers ? satisfactory ? gaps? Check they have not self-assessed inappropriately (DOPS, etc.).

7 **Session**: use the review button – printing out the page of professional competencies is useful. Review curriculum coverage.

8 Look at the forms together.

9 Link learning to competencies as a learning exercise together.

10 Comment on every competency area (ESR grading trainee against independent practice – CSR grading trainee against a standard at that stage of training).

11 Must end ST3 with competent entries.

12 CSA and AKT are independent assessments and do not guarantee any particular competency.

13 Enter the end of review period date (last day of current 6/12 post).

14 Check curriculum coverage.

15 Check skills log, i.e. forms validated.

16 Write some recommendations – particularly on the quality of evidence/ reflection. Are there any 'out of post' issues?

17 Be nurturing, informing, empowering, motivating and most of all encourage reflection.
18 Check OOH/CPR/AKT/CSA plans.
19 Submit via trainee.

CHAPTER 4

The e-portfolio and other curricular tools: how do trainers use curricular tools?

The map is not the territory. (Alfred Korzybski)

INTRODUCTION

Ten years ago the concept of curriculum in GP training was ill-defined, poorly understood and free-flowing. In this sense trainers and trainees were free to explore the territory but had no map or means of knowing where they'd been. The world moves on and, in an attempt to help the educational exploration, we now have the GP curriculum and its close neighbour the e-portfolio. Some argue that these tools are an attempt to define the indefinable: that they are restrictive and controlling. Others would argue that they are essential tools to ensure that the territory is well explored. We are still in the infancy of our experience with them.

This section briefly explores the concept of curriculum to help widen our appreciation, to offer a number of curriculum tools and to share wisdom on maximising the benefit of these new developments.

WHAT IS CURRICULUM?

How many definitions would you like? Most books on curriculum have at least a dozen, ranging from the simplistic 'Everything planned or guided by the particular institution' (Kerr J. *Changing the Curriculum*. London: University of London Press; 1968) to ones that define the aims, objectives, teaching methodologies, assessments and even the socio-political values underpinning the document (Bathory Z. Decentralisation issues in the introduction of new curriculum: the case of Hungary. *Prospects* 1986; XVI(1): 33–47).

Perhaps Hirst (*see* Hirst P. *Knowledge of the Curriculum*. London: Routledge; 1974) can help us out when he defines 'curriculum' as:

> . . . a programme of activities designed so that all participants will attain by learning certain specifiable ends or objectives . . . unless there is some point to planning the activities – some intended, learnable outcome, however vague – there is no such thing as curriculum.

So a curriculum should help both the trainer and the trainee develop some idea about where they are heading. We will look at some of the problems of using this sort of definition in a complex learning environment later but for now let's stick with what we've got.

For those of you with more academic interest in this, try Kelly A. *The Curriculum. Theory and Practice*. London: Paul Chapman Publishing; 1999, or even What is the curriculum?. In: Lawton D. *Social Change, Educational Theory and Curriculum Planning*. London: Routledge and Kegan Paul; 1973, or try looking for many of RM Harnden's publications in this area (often in the AMEE journal) or Prideaux D. ABC of learning and teaching in medicine: curriculum design. *BMJ*. 2003; **326**: 268–70.

The Scaling the Heights weblink at: http://resources.scalingtheheights.com/ identifies a number of other resources that have practical use – many of the regionally developed (Oxford, NW Thames and the IT Curriculum) resources are short enough and specific enough to be useful in particular teaching situations as well as informing personal development.

WHAT CURRICULUM RESOURCES HAVE WE GOT?
Principles
It is useful to remember some of the basics that underlie curriculum design.

Bloom's Taxonomy describes three domains and is a useful tool to help us identify and develop higher level function in trainees (*see* Table 4.1). The trainee and trainer can use the levels in each domain to widen and develop the educational experience and trainee's perception. The trainee can be encouraged to progress their thinking, enhance their attitudinal awareness and develop their skills base, in appropriate settings, down the scales. This should encourage a more in-depth approach to curriculum issues and stimulate higher quality portfolio entries.

Table 4.1

Cognitive	Affective	Psychomotor
Knowledge	Attitude	Skills
1 Recall data	1 Receive (awareness)	1 Imitation (copy)
2 Understand	2 Respond (react)	2 Manipulation (follow instructions)
3 Apply (use)	3 Value (understand and act)	3 Develop precision
4 Analyse (structure/ elements)	4 Organise personal value system	4 Articulation (combine, integrate related skills)
5 Synthesise (create/ build)	5 Internalise value system (adopt behaviour)	5 Naturalisation (automate, become expert)
6 Evaluate (assess, judge in relational terms)		

A revised version of the cognitive domain (Krathwol D. A revision of Bloom's Taxonomy: an overview. *Theory Into Practice* 2002; **41**(4)) that offers a structure for using this in teaching can be found at: www.unco.edu/cetl/sir/stating_outcome/documents/Krathwohl.pdf This reminds us that the curriculum is about a lot more than learning facts and perhaps the values against which we assimilate learning are the true foundations of the curriculum – ' the aim of education is the knowledge not of fact but of values'. Guilbert J. *Education Handbook for Health Personnel.* World Health Organization; 1997 has described the 'four Cs' of curriculum development.

➤ **Co-operation** – curriculum requires the combined input of learners, educators, the people doing the job and the assessors.
➤ **Continuous** – their needs to be a process for the curriculum to evolve.
➤ **Comprehensive** – the curriculum needs to be a tool that helps direct learners and educators. It needs to identify all the essential needs.
➤ **Concrete** – it needs to be specific.

This poses a real challenge to the curriculum developers in complex learning environments and places a responsibility on trainers to help learners navigate the challenges, particularly in areas where the curriculum is less well developed and defined.

WONCA (1997) suggested the following five-step process to help devise curricular statements.

1 Define the roles and tasks of the doctor within their setting.
2 Determine the required values, attitudes, skills and knowledge.
3 Clarify what needs to be done to acquire these attributes.
4 Determine how the trainer can assist in the process.
5 Determine how the learner will know when that has been achieved.

These steps seem to have a generic foundation that informs how trainers might approach learning in their own setting.

PRACTICAL TOOLS

This section aims to identify tools trainers are using in practice.

The RCGP curriculum

The development of this curriculum is arguably one of the boldest and most comprehensive educational developments for GPs anywhere in the world. Together with the College 'Blueprint' it forms an over-arching framework that guides trainees and educators towards the competencies of 'being a GP'.

It is a BIG concept! Not only does it set out to contain all the intended learning outcomes (ILOs) required to achieve competence as a GP but it also challenges us with new terminologies, a combination of domains (with sub-divisions), curriculum statements derived from these and matched to ILOs with a competency framework and defined assessments designed to integrate the whole system and provide the evidence, through the e-portfolio, for the Annual Review of Competency Progression (ARCP) panel to eventually award the Certificate of Completion of Training (CCT). Trainers admit to being a bit confused about how all this sits together, so a few definitions may help.

➤ *Core Curriculum Statement: Being a general practitioner*: this is the document that describes the roots, rationale and process that led to the curriculum at: www.rcgp-curriculum.org.uk/PDF/curr_1_Curriculum_Statement_Being_a_GP.pdf

➤ **Domains of competence**: the concept of 'being a GP' is then broken down into six domains of competence (*see* below) and three 'essential features' which can be applied contextually. These areas are subdivided for clarity. *See* www.rcgp-curriculum.org.uk/PDF/curr_1_Curriculum_Statement_Being_a_GP.pdf

THE RCGP DOMAINS OF COMPETENCE

'In order to demonstrate competence as a GP, the learner will need to acquire knowledge, skills and professional attitudes in a number of areas':
The Six Domains of core competences
1. Primary care management
2. Person-centred care
3. Specific problem-solving skills
4. A comprehensive approach
5. Community orientation
6. A holistic approach.
Essential features of the discipline of general practice
Three features are essential for a person-centred scientific discipline: *context, attitude and science.*
Essential Feature 1 – Contextual aspects
Essential Feature 2 – Attitudinal aspects
Essential Feature 3 – Scientific aspects
(Plus: Knowledge Base and Psychomotor Skills)

RCGP

➤ **Curriculum statements**: these are derived from the above domains and features and place these in defined learning areas with intended learning outcomes. It is argued that the domains and features may remain fixed as generic concepts but the statements will need to evolve. Curriculum statements can be found at: www.rcgp-curriculum.org.uk/rcgp_-_gp_curriculum_documents/gp_curriculum_statements.aspx

➤ **The MRCGP Competency Framework**: this framework maps the required competencies trainees need to demonstrate to the domains and features and also allows these competencies to then be mapped onto the various assessment and recording tools built into the curriculum – this will be dealt with in a separate chapter. *See* Table 4.2.

➤ **The e-portfolio**: The e-portfolio is a web-based tool that records details of achievement, documents all stages of training, and records evidence of workplace-based assessment (WPBA) and reviews with educational supervisors. Aspects of this will be covered in further chapters but the list below describes its scope.

- A record of all attachments.
- A record of clinical supervisors and educational supervisors.
- An educational log of educational activity.
- Logging this activity against RCGP curriculum statement headings.
- Educational supervisor logging this activity against professional competences.
- A message board for sending confidential messages.
- An unofficial system to make comments about progress and offer advice.
- A system to advertise meetings and courses to trainees across the region.
- A record of MRCGP examination attempts and passes.
- A record of WPBA forms.
- A record of CPR and AED certificate.
- A record of out-of-hours attendance.
- Personal development plan.
- Self-assessment of competence.
- Educational supervisors review of professional competencies.
- Review of educational reviews and annual review of competence progression.

MRCGP Competency Framework

Table 4.2

The curriculum	Related MRCGP competency areas
Primary care management	Clinical management
	Working with colleagues and in teams
	Primary care administration and information management and technology IM&T
Person-centred care	Communication and consulting skills

continued

The curriculum	Related MRCGP competency areas
Specific problem-solving skills	Data gathering and interpretation
	Making a diagnosis/making decisions
A comprehensive approach	Managing medical complexity
Community orientation	Community orientation
A holistic approach	Practicing holistically
Contextual features	Community orientation
Attitudinal features	Maintaining an ethical approach to practice
	Fitness to practise
Scientific features	Maintaining performance, learning and teaching

The GP curriculum and portfolio have understandably become the major tools in this area and we will look at trainers comments on these later. First we will look at other resources trainers are still finding useful in the 'post-MRCGP' world.

New Manchester Rating Scales

At: www.gp-training.net/training/assessment/formative/nmrs/index.htm These scales a bit dated now (1990s) but some trainers find them useful – the site contains 19 scales for use in clearly defined areas and is easily accessible online. The scales could be useful to help further dissect areas of identified learning need. These would have to be mapped onto the GP curriculum by the trainee.

New Northumberland Rating Scales

At: www.gp-training.net/training/tools/nnr.htm These scales were devised in the 1980s but have been updated through to 2006 – they are available as a spreadsheet that automatically scores trainee confidence levels in a wide range of areas and provide a useful way of assessing self-reported confidence across a wide spectrum of general practice activity.

The Wolverhampton Grid

This was an early attempt to design a comprehensive curriculum document – it is reproduced at www.radcliffepublishing.com/gptrainershandbook but is probably an outdated tool in comparison to the others mentioned – at least one trainer did mention it during our survey.

Initial educational planning list

At: www.radcliffepublishing.com/gptrainershandbook This is a short list that can be useful as an early planning guide towards the start of the training programme – it can help identify early priorities and is included as some practices have found it useful with medical student attachments.

OTHER RCGP RESOURCES

1 Ben Riley (one of the authors of the condensed curriculum guide) has produced a spreadsheet that can be used by trainees and educators. This spreadsheet automatically scores trainee self-reported confidence with the added benefit of being structured in line with the GP curriculum at: http://cms.rcgp.org.uk/gpcurriculum/docs/Condensed%20Curriculum%20 Guide%20-%20self-assessment%20scale.xls

2 The Learning and Teaching Guide Version3.2 (December 2008) at: www. rcgp-curriculum.org.uk/PDF/curr_The_Learning_and_Teaching_Guide_ dec08.pdf This guide is a useful overview of GP training. It highlights the following curriculum resources.

   - *e*-GP at: www.e-gp.org The RCGP's free new e-learning resource to support GP specialty training, featuring interactive e-learning modules covering the RCGP curriculum. Contains an e-learning module on *Being a General Practitioner* that introduces the core curriculum domains and essential application features. trainees can be signposted to particular modules.

   - RCGP InnovAiT at: www.rcgp-innovait.oxfordjournals.org The RCGP's monthly educational journal for associates in training, providing articles and AKT questions on general practice topics and curriculum-based issues. The journal is available to trainers for a special subscription rate of just £35. Throughout 2009, *InnovAiT* featured a series of articles on the new membership of the Royal College of General Practitioners (MRCGP) competences.

   - RCGP curriculum and assessment website at: www.rcgp-curriculum. org.uk Offers the latest news and information on GP training and the MRCGP. The documents section contains downloadable curriculum statements and the *Learning and Teaching Guide*.

   - RCGP curriculum map at: www.rcgp-curriculum.org.uk/extras/ curriculum The navigable online RCGP curriculum linking to online educational resources, and featuring a curriculum search engine. At the moment this site does not link to many educational resources but could prove an excellent resource if trainers use the facility to add their own experiences and resources.

   - RCGP curriculum and MRCGP books at: www.rcgp.org.uk/bookshop Order online at the RCGP bookstore for a 10% membership discount:

   - *The Condensed Curriculum Guide*: The official users' guide to the new RCGP curriculum and the MRCGP; for all GP specialty trainees, trainers and educators. It includes a condensed and indexed version of the official RCGP curriculum.

   - *General Practice Specialty Training: making it happen*: The RCGP guide for GP educators to the MRCGP assessments.

OTHER CURRICULAR RESOURCES
Good medical practice: GMC documentation

See at: www.gmc-uk.org/static/documents/content/GMC_GMP_0911.pdf Although this initiative was not primarily curriculum orientated the categories devised inevitably impinge on the concept of curriculum and, in a small number of categories, remind us of the scope of curriculum. The GMC site breaks each category down into descriptors:

➤ good clinical care
➤ maintaining good clinical care
➤ teaching and training
➤ relationship with patients
➤ working with colleagues
➤ relationships with patients
➤ health
➤ probity.

The European definition of general practice/family medicine

The GP curriculum is based on this WONCA definition:

> General practitioners/family doctors are specialist physicians trained in the principles of the discipline. They are personal doctors, primarily responsible for the provision of comprehensive and continuing care to every individual seeking medical care irrespective of age, sex and illness. They care for individuals in the context of their family, their community, and their culture, always respecting the autonomy of their patients. They recognise they will also have a professional responsibility to their community. In negotiating management plans with their patients they integrate physical, psychological, social, cultural and existential factors, utilising the knowledge and trust engendered by repeated contacts. General practitioners/family physicians exercise their professional role by promoting health, preventing disease and providing cure, care, or palliation. This is done either directly or through the services of others according to health needs and the resources available within the community they serve, assisting patients where necessary in accessing these services. They must take the responsibility for developing and maintaining their skills, personal balance and values as a basis for effective and safe patient care.

The link below defines 11 characteristics of the discipline related to 11 abilities that every specialist family doctor should master. Because of their interrelationship, they are clustered into six independent categories of core competence. These statements can form the basis of useful discussion with trainers and trainees at: www.woncaeurope.org/Web%20documents/European%20Definition%20 of%20family%20medicine/Definition%20EURACTshort%20version.pdf

There are a number of other historical resources that some trainers may find interesting.

➤ Fry J. *The Future General Practitioner.* London: RCGP; 1972 was ahead of its time and its 11 goals for GPs in training still have some relevance.

1 To develop an ability to make diagnoses which are expressed in physical, psychological and social terms simultaneously.
2 To recognise the patient as a unique individual and modify the ways in which they elicit data, make hypotheses and manage illness.
3 To develop an ability to make appropriate decisions about every presented problem.
4 To understand the way interpersonal relationships can affect the way illness occurs, presents and responds to treatment.
5 To develop an ability to understand and manage the use of time scales in a manner peculiar to general practice.
6 To acquire knowledge and skills in using the wide range of possible interventions.
7 To develop an understanding of the relationship between health and illness and the social characteristics of the patient.
8 To acquire knowledge of and skills in practice management.
9 To recognise the need for continuous medical education.
10 To acquire an understanding of basic research methods in practice.
11 To demonstrate ability and willingness to be self-critical.

➤ Pereira Gray DJ. *A System of Training for General Practice.* Occasional Paper 4. 2nd ed. London: Royal College of General Practitioners; 1979 adopted a reflective and patient-centred approach in defining the list of desired abilities in a trainee.

1 Knows what it feels like to be a patient.
2 Maintains the dignity of patients at all times.
3 Practices patient-centred medicine.
4 Identifies their own learning needs.
5 Remedies their own learning needs.
6 Assesses themselves objectively.
7 Accurately analyses their doctor/patient relationships.
8 Understands illness deeply as much in terms of the patient's behaviour as in pathological terms.
9 Assesses accurately the capacity of a home/household to care for a sick member.
10 Offers practical preventative advice (even suggesting in more than 50% of cases).
11 Tolerates uncertainty.
12 Promotes patient autonomy.
13 Reads and critically assesses the literature in general practice.

14 Feels a responsibility for the health of their registered patients.

15 Can analyse a problem, devise a research project, carry it out and present the results.

Specific sub-curriculum lists

Trainers identified a number of resources in specific areas.

➤ **The IT list** – this is an NHS defined aspiration list for desired IT skills for all health professionals at: www.resources.scalingtheheights.com/ it_learning_expectations.htm

➤ **The leadership curriculum** – this is a recently devised curriculum to guide the emerging clinical leadership agenda:
  - demonstrating personal qualities – doctors showing effective leadership need to draw upon their values, strengths, and abilities to deliver high standards of care
  - developing self-awareness
  - managing yourself
  - continuing personal development
  - acting with integrity.

➤ **Working with others** – doctors show leadership by working with others in teams and networks to deliver and improve services:
  - developing networks
  - building and maintaining relationships
  - encouraging contribution
  - working within teams.

➤ **Improving services** – doctors showing effective leadership are focused on the success of the organisation in which they work:
  - planning
  - managing resources
  - managing people
  - managing performance.

➤ **Setting direction** – doctors showing effective leadership contribute to the strategy and aspirations of the organisation and act in a manner consistent with its values:
  - identifying the contexts for change
  - applying knowledge and evidence
  - making decisions
  - evaluating impact.

➤ **Difficult lists** – this list was produced by a registrar group:
  - termination request
  - contraception in general
  - tired all the time presentations
  - angry and critical patients

- the non-urgent 'extra'
- patients 'demanding' a certain treatment
- depressed patients
- headaches.

➤ **Admitting you are wrong/don't know what's wrong** – a survey of GPs in Canada (in the UBC handbook) revealed the following common issues that trainees struggled with:
- achieving concordance
- dealing with diagnostic uncertainty
- achieving appropriate follow-up
- failure of or absence of any treatment
- inadequate resources
- personal emotional reactions
- time management
- too many patients
- keeping up to date
- knowing when to intervene and when not to
- dealing with waiting lists
- dealing with patients expectations
- sharing understanding with patients.

➤ **The law and ethics curriculum** – this shortlist highlights the major areas in this field:
- informed consent (including capacity)
- the clinical relationship (truth, trust and communication)
- confidentiality
- medical research
- human reproductive issues
- the new genetics
- children
- mental disorders
- life, death, dying and killing
- vulnerability created by the duties of a doctor
- resource allocation
- rights and responsibilities.

➤ **Forms you should know** – self-explanatory, really. However, in the IT age many of these functions are now computer-based (*see* Table 4.3).

Table 4.3

Prescription forms – computer and hand-written	Yellow card system
Fitness for work form	Prescription exemption form
Private sick notes	DEA form
Non-NHS prescriptions	Wheelchair forms

continued

Practice associated documentation	Vaccination forms
Referral forms/templates/proforma	RTA documentation
Registration forms	Investigation forms
Cremation forms	Complaint forms
Death certificates	Significant event forms
Insurance forms	HGV forms
DS 1500	Taxi forms
Seat belt exemptions	Occupational health forms
Legal reports	(CAA, diving, etc.)
Insurance reports	Mat B1
Abortion Act documentation	
DLA forms	
DWP reports	
DVLA reports	

➤ **Need to know list** – this list is designed to help a new trainee prioritise their needs in the first weeks.
   Priority 1
   - the computer system – accessing appointments, looking at essential records, recording notes, accessing internet, basic template use
   - calling a patient
   - initiating investigations
   - referring patients
   - writing a prescription
   - the repeat prescribing system
   - other essential 'idiosyncratic' practice systems
   - accessing support
   - basic portfolio use.
   Priority 2
   - visits system
   - use of PHCT
   - wider appreciation of IT use
   - wider use of PHCT and other resources
   - wider use of in-house resources
   - wider awareness of educational need and resources.
   Priority 3
   - on call systems
   - financial systems
   - practice policies
   - audit systems
   - practice management awareness

   – complaints systems
   – development of PDP.
➤ **The Stamford 25** – this is an interesting list of 25 procedures that are seen as appropriate competencies for US internal medicine trainees and, with the advent of near patient testing and transfer of care to primary care, may be a challenge for future of primary care educators.
1 Fundoscopic exam, papilledema, etc. using panoptic and regular ophthalmoscopes.
2 Pupillary responses and relevant anatomy.
3 Thyroid exam technique.
4 Examination of neck veins/JVP for both level (volume) and common abnormal wave forms; tricuspid regurgitation (ventricularisation of 'v' waves); canon 'a' waves, etc.
5 Lung: surface anatomy, percussion technique, finding upper border of liver dullness, finding Traube's space.
6 Evaluation of parasternal heave, and other precordial movements.
7 Examination of the liver.
8 Palpation, percussion of spleen.
9 Evaluation of common gait abnormalities.
10 The ankle jerk: if performed in a recumbent patient, one must have the right technique for each of the reflexes.
11 Stigmata of liver disease from head to foot: be able to list, identify, and demonstrate.
12 Internal capsule stroke: list, identify, and demonstrate common physical findings: lower facial weakness, distal motor weakness, hyperreflexia, absent abdominal reflex on that side, abnormal plantar (Babinski) and abnormal tone, etc.
13 Knee exam.
14 Cardiac second sounds: splitting, wide splitting and paradoxical splitting.
15 Evaluation of involuntary movements such as tremors, etc.
16 The hand in diagnosis: recognise clubbing, cyanosis, other common nail and hand findings.
17 The tongue in diagnosis.
18 Shoulder exam (specifically testing rotator cuff tears, ac joint, etc.).
19 Blood pressure assessment (this is more technique-driven than health care workers realise), pulsus paradoxus assessment.
20 Cervical lymph node assessment.
21 Ascites detection and abdominal venous patterns.
22 Rectal exam.
23 Evaluation of scrotal mass – differential between hydrocele, varicocele, spermatocele, testicular mass, etc.

24 Cerebellar testing.

25 Bedside ultrasound.

Summary

This section has offered resources related to the concept of curriculum – many of these are related to the GP curriculum and the portfolio but others expand our perspective and challenge us as trainers to use a variety of tools to address the learning needs of our trainees. In the next section we will look at the advice trainers have to help us use these tools effectively.

WHAT TIPS CAN TRAINERS OFFER ON HOW TO MAKE THE PORTFOLIO EFFECTIVE IN TRAINING?

Most of the advice trainers offered here was essentially related to the process of using the portfolio and curriculum. Both trainer and trainee need to familiarise themselves with the structural elements of the e-system and there is no substitute for spending time exploring the system. Trainers suggested an early tutorial with the trainee taking the lead and demonstrating the portfolio to the trainer with both parties sharing knowledge and experience. The rest of this section structures the advice trainers thought most helpful.

➤ **From the start:** start early . . . review entries regularly (at least twice a week) – 'nag' incessantly!

➤ **Encouraging quality entries:**

For the trainee – do a tutorial on reflective practice (*see* the section on WPBA in Chapter 3), avoid simple event descriptions, encourage a range of evidence, encourage the recording of contextual application of learning, encourage a critical approach, encourage justification of approach, encourage evidence of development in record, encourage record of use of feedback in all stages of learning, encourage collection of 'naturally occurring evidence', i.e. that occurring from day to day across the whole spectrum of experience.

For the clinical supervisor and educational supervisor – reference any comments to the portfolio, justify any comments, give developmental feedback, show awareness of 'feedback rules' (*see* Chapter 3), give feedback on current level of attainment, comment on strengths and weaknesses, help formulate a PDP (*see* the section on PDP quality in Chapter 4), critically evaluate evidence and offer advice on how needs might be met, triangulate evidence if possible, offer advice on how to improve portfolio record.

➤ **Adopt a 'sharing' approach:** encourage shared entries, review entries/ PDP/diary dates, etc. – one trainer suggested using the clinical record system to keep contemporaneous notes on a daily basis by setting the trainee up as a temporary resident!

➤ **Other 'process' advice:** identify 'rare' competencies (i.e. teaching, mentoring, genetics, maintaining professionalism) and plan how to address them, do 'little and often'. Try to be as specific as possible, achieve early out-of-hours involvement, use the messaging system to liaise with the trainee and other trainers and supervisors (particularly if you have any doubts), plan a calendar to set targets.

Trainers emphasised that trainees need to satisfactory completion and entry quality as their responsibility.

Bradford VTS have an excellent set of advice sheets covering the use of the curriculum and portfolio at: www.bradfordvts.co.uk/ED_SUPERVISION/ tipsforTrainees.htm This website is a 'must-search' resource for trainees and trainers with resources covering all areas of GP training.

Other resources for trainers in this area include:

➤ The RCGP Learning and Teaching Guide at: www.rcgp-curriculum.org.uk/ PDF/curr_The_Learning_and_Teaching_Guide_dec08.pdf
➤ A brief RCGP guide to Clinical Supervision at: www.westmidlandsdeanery. nhs.uk/LinkClick.aspx?fileticket=2Zf9yHHuSvg%3d&tabid=170&mid=898
➤ The West Midland Deanery Site has some useful advice and other links at: www.westmidlandsdeanery.nhs.uk/GeneralPractice/Trainers/ ClinicalSupervision.aspx

THE PERSONAL DEVELOPMENT PLAN

Personal development plans (PDPs) are seen as underpinning continuing medical education in almost all of the healthcare sector. Trainers are advised to support trainees in the development of their PDPs and the quality of the latter is reported to vary somewhat.

What are PDPs?

In the UK, the QAA (2004) define PDP as:

> Personal Development Planning is a structured and supported process undertaken by an individual to reflect upon their own learning, performance and/or achievement and to plan for their personal, educational and career development. The primary objective for PDP is to improve the capacity of individuals to understand what and how they are learning, and to review, plan and take responsibility for their own learning, helping students:
> ➤ become more effective, independent and confident self-directed learners;
> ➤ understand how they are learning and relate their learning to a wider context;
> ➤ improve their general skills for study and career management;

➤ articulate personal goals and evaluate progress towards their achievement;
➤ and encourage a positive attitude to learning throughout life.

Wojtczak (Wojtczak A. Glossary of medical education terms: Part 1. *Medical Teacher*. 2002; 24(2): 216–19) defines a PDP in the context of medical education as:

> A list of educational needs, development goals and actions and processes, compiled by learners and used in systematic management and periodic reviews of learning. It is an integral part of reflective practice and self-directed learning for professionals. It can be equally valuable in teacher-directed medical training for maintaining learner-centred approaches and shared objectives. PDP can be used to manage learning needs systematically, to set development and performance improvement goals, organise learning activities and review outcomes. Some educational organisations accept completed plans for accredited professional development and health managers link them with appraisals.

PDPs are underpinned by a number of processes:
➤ critical appraisal
➤ self-awareness
➤ reflective practice
➤ learning skills
➤ motivation
➤ resource awareness
➤ adult learning
➤ real life grounding
➤ evidence-based.

Trainers recommended an early discussion on this area – perhaps sharing examples of PDPs. trainers did not mention any specific books in this area; however, a recognised publication is available: Rughani A. *The GP's Guide to PDPs*. 2nd ed. Oxford: Radcliffe Medical Press; 2001.

A simple tool to assess a PDP quality is shown in the appendix and is also available at: www.radcliffepublishing.com/gptrainershandbook

SUMMARY

Trainers are acutely aware that their role is to facilitate the development of the next generation of doctors. All of our systems are designed to help achieve this, and they are all flawed! The challenge for trainers and trainees is to navigate the territory maximising the use of the various 'maps' available. The backwash effect of the MRCGP and the high-stakes nature of the portfolio inevitably dominate the educational experience and we are still in the infancy of our experience with this system. This section offers a range of curricular tools that can be used too widen our perspectives.

Figure 4.1 demonstrates how any curriculum has to achieve a sort of balance and helps us understand some of the effects of a high-definition curriculum. A number of years ago Roger Neighbour identified the 14 hallmarks of the 'Excellent registrar' (*see* Table 4.4).

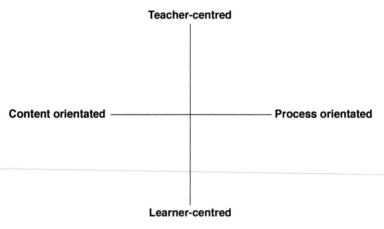

Figure 4.1: Curriculum orientation.

Table 4.4 The 14 hallmarks of the Excellent registrar

Positive response to novelty	Genuine caring with respect for people
Good clinical competence	Good self-awareness
Good group skills	Good personal qualities (undefined)
High educability (undefined)	Strong motivation
A balanced lifestyle/personality	Industrious
Good communication skills	A sense of mission
Good critical abilities	Good diversity of approach

Shaw, Moxham and Cairns (Shaw CJ, Moxham VF, Cairns H. *Managing the Take*, available at: http://careers.bmj.com/careers/advice/view-article.html?id=20000896) contains a summary of the social and cognitive skills that lead to improved performance:

    Social Skills:
➤ Communication
➤ Information sharing
➤ Feedback

➤ Leadership
➤ Team building

Cognitive Skills:

➤ Preparation and Planning
➤ Workload management
➤ Prioritisation and allocation
➤ Monitoring and Recognition
➤ Situational awareness
➤ Decision-making
➤ Re-evaluation

These two lists challenge us as trainers: How can I help develop these attributes in my trainees? How do these qualities relate to the portfolio and its requirements? It challenges trainers to look for 'deep meaningful learning' and avoid superficial 'tick-box' training. Marshall wrote: 'Education must have an end in view as it is not an end in itself.' Trainers are ideally placed to encourage the appropriate ends.

Appendix

PERSONAL DEVELOPMENT PLAN ASSESSMENT TOOL

Mentor...

Learner..

Date...

AREA OF ASSESSMENT

	Not covered	Adequate coverage	Excellent coverage

➤ **Learning needs assessed**
Uses a range of techniques to assess learning needs that cover knowledge, skills and attitudes. These are stated clearly and specifically, are prioritised and show insight

➤ **Learning plan**
This is appropriate, varied, achievable, time-lined, described in adequate detail and addresses the needs, environment and learning preferences of the learner

➤ **Assessment of learning**
This covers planned outcomes, a plan for assessing outcomes with an appropriate range of methods

➤ **The learning activity**
This is recorded and evidenced

➤ **Meaning**
There is a record of deep covering the learning outcomes in relation to the assessed outcomes and future needs. The reflection covers issues of knowledge, skills and attitudes as well as reflection on learning strategies

➤ **Evidence of learning**
There is evidence of appropriate assessment of the application of new learning, i.e. in performance

➤ **Evidence of continuity of learning**
There is evidence that the range of new learning is integrated with past learning and used in future planning

➤ **Overall assessment of quality**

Comments

CHAPTER 5

Tutorials: how do trainers plan tutorials?

*It is always wise to look ahead but difficult to
look farther than you can see
(Winston Churchill)*

INTRODUCTION

Many of the tools mentioned throughout this manual are designed to be used in a tutorial setting. So what is this section about? This section describes how trainers performed two tasks. First: How did they plan the format of the tutorial? And, secondly: How did they find out if the tutorial 'worked'? The section finishes with an overview of tutorial planning.

Trainers should ask themselves a critical question at this point: 'When do I learn best?' The answer seems to lie in four main areas:

➤ when I need to: i.e. when I am aware of it and its relevance
➤ when I want to: i.e. when both the atmosphere and my attitude is suitable
➤ when I can: i.e. when the opportunity and the situation allow it
➤ when it works: i.e. I see its value and it integrates with my established learning.

Trainers need to apply the practicalities of these points. Tutorials need to be relevant (sometimes difficult because they can be perceived as detached from the clinical core of the work) and jointly agreed. The trainer and trainee must create a suitable environment and feel positive about the potential for learning. The time should be protected, valued and 'seized'. *Carpe diem* (seize the day) encapsulates the concept that learning opportunities can be fleeting moments and should be grasped firmly as they arise – again, difficult to achieve in the protected-time tutorial. Trainers need to look for these moments from day to day and patient to patient. Trainers need to create the environment where the value of new learning can be tested and proved. Finally, trainers now need to help the trainee translate the learning achieved and the learning needs identified into entries on the e-portfolio and PDP. These points are the challenge to trainers as they plan the tutorial programme.

TUTORIAL STRUCTURE

The trainers' approach

Many trainers have evolved their own tutorial assessment scales. An analysis of these reveals a number of commonalties.

1 A subject area was identified jointly.
2 Aims and objectives in this area were jointly negotiated (often in relation to curriculum competencies or the needs of WPBA).
3 The method to tackle these aims was negotiated with enjoyment high on the agenda.
4 The timing, setting and facilitator were agreed.
5 The process occurred.
6 The trainee was asked for feedback in six areas:
   - relevance
   - whether aims were achieved, and what was learnt
   - what worked well?
   - what could have been better?
   - enjoyment
   - need for follow-up work.
7 The feedback was jointly reviewed.
8 The event was related to the e-portfolio.

The forms varied in their design: some were purely feedback and others combined this with a recording function and acted as an event record. The frequency of use of these forms seems to have declined markedly in the face of the demands of the e-portfolio. See at: www.radcliffepublishing.com/gptrainers handbook for some examples of forms in use.

The assessors' approach

Many regions actively assessed trainers' teaching skills – often using videos of tutorials. It appear this practice has also decreased and there may be a need to re-explore this area. The most common approach was the video assessment of a tutorial and in some areas this was, and might again be, a compulsory component of re-approval for training.

Does the process used for this assessment help us plan the tutorial – maybe! It will *definitely* help trainers produce a reasonable video of the tutorial and this *may* improve the learning process.

Two models of the tutorial process are discussed by Ruscoe M. Assessment of the tutorial. *Education for General Practice*. 1994; 5: 260–8, describing a task and a process analysis. These are shown in Tables 5.1 and 5.2.

The major concept these models add to the trainer-based approach is the idea of 'baggage checking'. This is the tutorial equivalent of housekeeping. It

Table 5.1 Task orientated model of tutorial

1	Learner needs jointly identified
2	Learning need discussed
3	Learning need agreed
4	Teaching strategy proposed
5	Teaching strategy agreed
6	Teaching strategy implemented
7	Future needs identified
8	Future needs discussed
9	Future needs agreed

Table 5.2 Process model of tutorial

1	Introduction
2	Baggage check
3	Exploration
4	Discovery
5	Planning
6	Evaluation

is useful to highlight the need to resolve any outstanding personal, clinical or educational demands that would impede the learning process *before* you start. The process model also highlights the issue of planning and emphasises that the tutorial is part of a process and should not be seen in isolation.

The qualitative aspects of teaching also come under scrutiny by the assessors. These can be looked at under a number of headings.

1 **Structural** – does the training happen in a good environment in protected time?
2 **Process** – is the process learner-centred, flexible, sensitive and stimulating?
3 **Outcomes** – are these sought and considered maturely? How do they relate to the e-portfolio?

The whole process should occur in the context of an appropriate trainer/trainee relationship. *See* www.radcliffepublishing.com/gptrainershandbook for an assessment form combining these points.

STYLE

All trainers teach in style – of course they do? But *what* style? Heron produced a description of different facilitation styles that could be adopted by trainers as they performed various tasks. This model challenges the trainer to assess whether they use the appropriate style consistently.

He describes three modes of facilitation each usable in six dimensions producing the grid shown in Table 5.3.

Table 5.3 Facilitation

Dimensions	Hierarchical	Modes Co-operative	Autonomous
Planning Setting objectives and assessments	Trainer plans but does not really negotiate	Trainer negotiates and co-ordinates	Trainer delegates
Meaning Making sense of and understanding the task and process of learning	Trainer inputs theory, interprets and assesses	Trainer asks neutral questions reflection (what is happening now?), uses descriptive feedback and negotiates assessment	Trainer uses reflection Group self-assesses and self-analyses
Confronting Raising awareness about learning blocks and blocks in enabling self-confrontation	Trainer interprets and may even describe block	Trainer describes events and asks for views on avoidance	Trainer provides safe environment
Feeling Identify negative emotional processes, interrupt them and alter them. Achieving a balance of emotions	Trainer decides how feelings are managed and thinks for the group. Trainer gives permission for catharsis	Trainer works with the group to develop ways to cope with feelings	Trainer gives space to manage feelings
Structuring Giving form to the learning process	Trainer takes over the design and supervision	Trainer co-operates to let rules emerge using counselling	Trainer delegates design skills
Valuing Creating climate of respect	Trainer uses actions and commitment, i.e. charisma. Trainer has positive regard for others	Trainer collaborates to allow self-respect and favourable climate to emerge	Trainer lets the group determine its own climate. Makes self-disclosures on values

Some trainers adopt a very hierarchical approach to structuring, a co-operative approach to valuing and an autonomous one to confronting. The model challenges trainers to consider the appropriate style for each situation.

Quirk describes four types of teaching style.

1 **Assertive-style teaching**: extrovert and tends to direct the process by leading from the front.
2 **Suggestive-style teaching**: tends to offer ideas and thoughts readily.
3 **Collaborative-style teaching**: identifies and legitimises the learners difficulties.
4 **Facilitative-style teaching**: encourages the learner to discover the way forward using and developing their own skills.

The model can be interpreted to imply that all good trainers use a facilitative style. Even if it is accepted as an ideal, this style will be ineffective and inappropriate in some situations. The under-confident trainee may need the trainer to give an answer before feeling able to offer their own; many trainees will face situations where they can see no options and require prompting with a range of suggestions. In these situations it may be ideal to encourage the trainee to develop their confidence or research the problem – but trainers have to operate in the real world where confidence is not built up overnight and patients can't wait 30 minutes while the trainee looks something up! The models can help trainers become more aware of the style options and increase their repertoire of options.

The spectrum of approach is illustrated by the 'fathers' of adult learning and directed or systematic instruction. Knowles's theory of andragogy is an attempt to develop a theory specifically for adult learning. Knowles emphasises that adults are self-directed and expect to take responsibility for decisions – any teaching must take this into account. Andragogy makes the following assumptions about the design of learning.

1 Adult learners need to know why they need to learn something.
2 Adults learners need to learn experientially.
3 Adults approach learning as problem-solving.
4 Adults learn best when the topic is of immediate value.

(Knowles MS. *The Modern Practice of Adult Education: andragogy versus pedagogy.* Englewood Cliffs: Prentice Hall/Cambridge; 1970, 1980.)

In practical terms, this means that trainers need to focus more on the process and less on the content being taught. Strategies such as case studies, role playing, simulations and self-evaluation are most useful. Trainers adopt a role of facilitator or resource rather than lecturer or grader.

However: 'For every theory there is an equal and opposite theory' and Gagne's book, *The Conditions of Learning*, first published in 1965 (Gagne R. *The Conditions of Learning*. 4th ed. New York: Holt, Rinehart & Winston; 1985) outlines a more systematic approach. His nine steps are described in Table 5.4.

These theories offer a range of approaches for trainers – the optimal approach will vary depending on the learner (how self-motivating and capable are they as learners?), the learning objectives (are they fairly specific or even task orientated or are they more exploratory?) and the trainer (how aware is the trainer? How self-confident is the trainer?).

Table 5.4 Gagne's instructional events

Instructional event	Internal mental process
1 Gain attention	Stimuli activate receptors
2 Inform learners of objectives	Creates level of expectation for learning
3 Stimulate recall of prior learning	Retrieval and activation of short-term memory
4 Present the content	Selective perception of content
5 Provide 'learning guidance'	Semantic encoding for storage in long-term memory
6 Elicit performance (practice)	Responds to questions to enhance encoding and verification
7 Provide feedback	Reinforcement and assessment of correct performance
8 Assess performance	Retrieval and reinforcement of content as final evaluation
9 Enhance retention and transfer to the job	Retrieval and generalisation of learned skill to new situation

THEORY

> These are my principles and if you don't like them, I have others. (Anon)

When trainers were asked 'Is educational theory useful?', the most common response was 'NO!'. Just like Julia in Coetzee's 'Summertime' they believe 'pragmatism always beats principles; that's just the way things are'. On the basis of 'no pain – no gain', *some* trainers found *some* of the theory useful. This section is a brief description of which bits, where and how. Give it a read and who knows?

Role modelling, apprenticeship and coaching

Even within the English-speaking Western world, training systems for primary care physicians are incredibly variable. The common themes seem to be role modelling, apprenticeship and coaching. The most influential, stimulating and exciting training programmes will ultimately rise or fall depending on the individuals whom learners can role model themselves upon.

Descriptions of excellent learning environments stress the presence of good role models. Most doctors have little problem naming at least one influential role model in their own education. These people have often demonstrated mastery in a particular area. They have usually combined this with *caritas* and the feeling of contentment derived from a job well done. Each learner models themselves on a variety of individuals to a variable degree and much of this learning is at the unconscious level for both the learner and the role model. The trainer can attempt to influence this process in a number of ways: by raising awareness in the learner and trainers that this process is at work to try and move the experience into the conscious sphere; highlighting the positive features of a particular role model; highlighting the negative features of a particular role model to avoid poor role modelling and attempt to create counterpoint features for modelling; consciously exposing the learner to role models who demonstrate attributes the learner (and/or trainer) perceives as their own educational needs. These observations and the attributes of the ideal primary care physician (*see* Tables 5.5 and 5.6 below – lists derived from research based

Table 5.5 The attributes of the ideal primary care physician (after Battles *et al.*)

Communication skills	Relationships with patients	Personal attributes	Professional attitudes
1. Can communicate	1. Demonstrates care and concern	1. Empathic and understanding	1. Competent
2. Is a good listener	2. Interested in patients	2. Has common sense	2. Compassionate
3. Has professional respect for individual worth regardless of social status, moral values, economic status or lifestyle	3. Accepts different patients	3. Honesty	
	4. Patient	4. Has integrity	4. Respectful
	5. Has rapport with patients	5. Courteous	5. Confident
	6. Has empathy for families	6. Sensitive	6. Flexible
	7. Comforting	7. Possesses wisdom	7. Comprehensive
	8. Uses self-restraint	8. Optimistic	8. Persistent
	9. Compulsive	9. Supportive	9. Humble
	10. Willing to and able to work in a team	10. Can formulate goals and ways to meet them	10. Accepts own mortality
		11. Firm	11. Interested in human nature enjoying the beauty in each person
		12. Shows love	12. Curious and keeps up to date
		13. Tolerant	

on patient and professional viewpoints) represent a challenge to trainers and to those who approve training practices. Whilst it may be possible to increase trainee awareness of these desirable qualities the apprenticeship model illustrates that the qualities actually observed and experienced will be more influential.

Table 5.6 The 'ideal' qualities of a GP: what patients want from their GP

Factor 1 Communication: illness experience, communication and doctor-patient relationship
Deal with my worries about the problem
Listen to everything I have to say about my problem
Be interested in what I want to know
Understand my main reason for coming
Be friendly and approachable
Make me feel really understood
Find out how serious my problem is
Clearly explain what the problem is
Clearly explain what should happen

Factor 2 Partnership: interest in beliefs, expectations and negotiating common ground
Be interested in what I think the problem is
Discuss and agree with me what the problem is
Be interested in what I want done
Be interested in what treatment I want
Discuss and agree with me on treatment

Factor 3 Health promotion:
Give advice on how to reduce the risk of future illness
Give advice on how to stay healthy in the future

Other aspects of consultation desired:
Examine me fully
Give me a prescription when I want one
Give advice on what I can do
Understand my emotional needs
Be interested in how the problem affects my life

The stages of apprenticeship offer some insights for the training practice:

I   Observation: apprentices observe – warts and all! They see things go well and not so well.
II Modelling: without any other input the apprentice starts to model their behaviour on what they observe. At this stage they cannot reliably identify which behaviours are most desirable. (Think of how young children often demonstrate the parent's most irritating habits!)

III Articulation: the trainer describes how to perform the skill. The apprentice questions and demonstrates understanding at the verbal level.
IV Demonstration: the trainer demonstrates the process to the apprentice; the apprentice demonstrates the process, with support and protection to the trainer.
V Withdrawal: the trainer slowly withdraws under control.
VI Independence: the apprentice has acquired independent skill.
VII Generalising: the trainer encourages the apprentice to analyse new skills, develop principles and use these to solve new problems.
VIII Coaching: the trainer encourages the accomplished apprentice to identify areas and techniques for possible refinement.

(Coaching is the process of enhancing the performance and learning ability of others, using motivation, effective questioning, feedback and personality style awareness techniques.)
This process describes how trainees learn many new skills. Often the learning has an implicit element and trainers are using these concepts subconsciously (unconscious competence – *see* later section). An explicit awareness can be helpful if problem situations arise (poor role modelling) or a particular problem emerges (attach the anxious trainee to the most relaxed partner?).

Johari's window

This is a pictorial model that aims to aid understanding of where change might occur. It is shown in Figure 5.1.

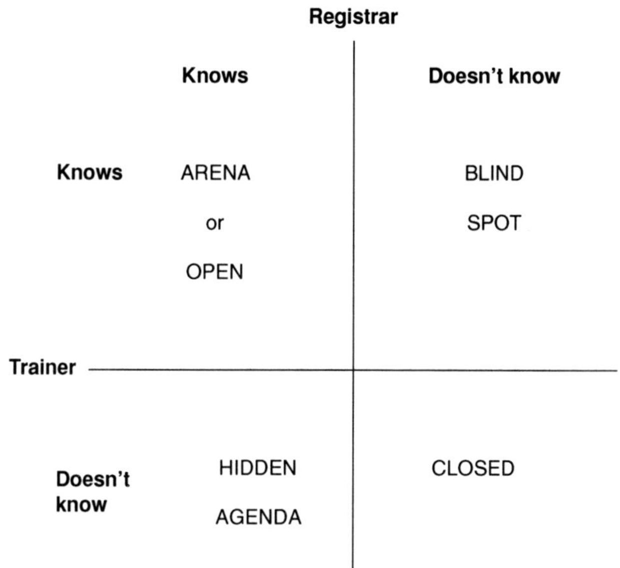

Figure 5.1: Johari window.

The theory states that you learn more as you open up the arena. You do this by reducing the blind spot and the hidden agenda. As the axes move you necessarily reduce the closed area too. So what does that mean in practical terms? This tool is useful to convey your philosophy of training to the 'theorist' type trainee, particularly if you feel there is an element of reticence in giving and receiving feedback. In practical terms it encourages positive attitudes to self-disclosure and feedback.

Competency model

This is a model to describe the process of learning a new skill. It is shown in Figure 5.2.

1– UNCONSCIOUS   2– CONSCIOUS
INCOMPETENCE   COMPETENCE

3– CONSCIOUS   4– UNCONSCIOUS
INCOMPETENCE   COMPETENCE

Figure 5.2: The competency model.

The theory holds that we move from unconscious incompetence to unconscious competence. It is helpful in a number of ways:
➤ it reminds trainees that new skills are just over the horizon
➤ it reminds trainees that they have unconsciously competent skills already
➤ it highlights that the process of learning includes a period of conscious incompetence, i.e. they are going to feel uncomfortable and if they don't something is wrong!
➤ it reminds trainers that to teach something it helps to be consciously competent to some degree (and also that they too have unconscious incompetence!).

The educational triangle

Figures 5.3 and 5.4 show the educational triangle in two forms. The first is the conventional model and the second emphasises the processes involved. Many trainees come into general practice with years of didactic, ritually humiliating educational experience. Some of the approaches GP trainers use are completely novel to them. They have acquired all sorts of educational myths, i.e. 'all assessment is summative and I must produce the right answers' or 'admitting you don't know is a sign of weakness'. It helps to give them insight to the formative nature of the process. This can be done simply with a diagram (for the visual learner), as a discussion (perhaps for the reflector) or you can make a series of

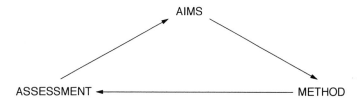

Figure 5.3: The conventional educational cycle.

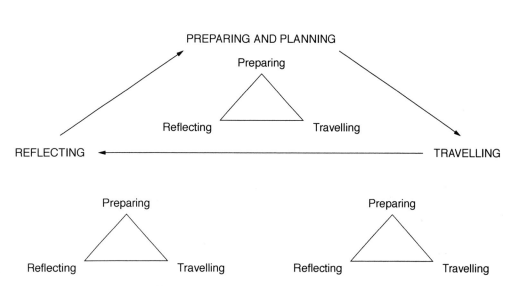

Figure 5.4: The process educational cycle: wheels within wheels.

cards and play with them on the floor (for the activist). It is helpful to point out that each element of the process-type educational triangle has its own internal triangle also – even make a set of smaller cards to illustrate the point.

The cycle is more accurately described as a spiral and this concept helps to reinforce that we all get second, third, fourth and perhaps limitless opportunities to learn as problems re-present. This gives us the dual opportunities of reinforcing past learning and looking for more insights in the light of that learning.

This type of exercise can significantly alter a trainee's attitude to the learning process.

Field dependence model

This is a model of learning styles developed by Riding and Cheema (1991). It contains a number of concepts but the field dependency idea can have practical value. The characteristics of field dependent/independent types are shown in Table 5.7.

Table 5.7

Field dependent learners	Field independent learners
Relate to peers well	Require little interaction with peers
Use external frames of reference	Use internal frame of reference
Need external reinforcement	Intrinsic reinforcement
Need structured work	Structure own learning needs
Good interpersonal skills	Need help in developing social skills
Need help problem solving	Good at problem solving

If the trainer can recognise their trainee's field dependency then it can be used to design appropriate facilitation methods. It is also useful for trainers to identify their own field dependency preferences (*see* Table 5.8).

Table 5.8

Field dependent teachers	Field independent teachers
Prefer interaction with learners	Prefer formal approaches
Are reluctant to express criticism	Emphasise their own standards
Are concerned with a positive atmosphere	Focus on content rather than attitudes or ambience

Hemispheric dominance theory (after Sperry, Gregorac, Butler and Hermann)

This theory holds that one side of our brain has a controlling dominance over some aspects of our thinking and behaviour. In McCarthy B. *The Hemispheric Mode Indicator: Right and Left Brain Approaches to Learning.* Barrington, IL: Excel; 1993, a technique is described to identify an individuals bias. Many feel this can be assessed just as readily by observation (*see* Table 5.9):

Table 5.9

RIGHT DOMINANT	creative, musical, rhythmical, intuitive, spontaneous
LEFT DOMINANT	logical, organised, rational, controlled, deductive

Teaching methods can then be tailored to fit the preferred instructional mode of the trainee. This concept is illustrated further and is also available at www. radcliffepublishing.com/gptrainershandbook

Other points to note

Communication

It has been said that input into the human brain occurs in the proportions set out in Table 5.10:

Table 5.10

A	Sight	7%	A major input and major distraction
B	Sound	20%	
C	Touch	5%	
D	Taste/smell	5%	

Another interesting variation of this (attributed to Glasser) is that most people learn:

10%	of what they read
20%	of what they hear
30%	of what they see
50%	of what they see AND hear
70%	of what they talk over with others
80%	of what they use and do in real life
90%	of what they teach to someone else.

It is a commonly quoted 'fact' that 60% of communication is at the non-verbal level. So demonstration, peer discussion/interaction, multimodal material and non-verbal communication skills are vitally important in teaching. Messages can be reinforced by combining visual, auditory, sensual and affective inputs. This principle of 'linkage' seems to increase the likelihood of retention of learning. The ability of the brain to store and retrieve information is increased if the learning is 'linked' to almost any other input: the more links the better (to a degree), i.e. try and link learning to patients, places, times, feelings, diseases, sounds, sights, smells, tastes, etc. and using the learners preferences may improve the efficiency of the process. If nothing else it should make the learning process varied and fun! Perhaps the most important link to consider is how new learning integrates with established learning – anchoring new learning to previous learning is a powerful process.

Key phrases
These five phrases can act as a simple aide-memoir in tutorials. trainers should encourage the trainee to move from:
➤ the unknown to the known
➤ the concrete to the abstract
➤ the whole to the parts
➤ the simple to the complex
➤ the general to the specific.

Problem-solving styles
One of the core skills of general practice is the ability to problem solve efficiently. How can trainers teach this? A clue may lie in the individual's problem-

solving style. Cox and Ewan described three styles (Cox KR and Ewan CE, editors, *The Medical Teacher*. Edinburgh: Churchill Livingstone; 1982).

Pattern recognition

Much of our clinical training and experience results in an internalised data-bank of clinical patterns. This recognition system seems to be active in the first few minutes of a consultation. If a pattern is not recognised within this time then it probably won't be at all. Pattern recognition requires knowledge and experience but the trainer can try to imprint patterns on the trainee by highlighting them when seen and raising awareness of the pattern recognition system. One area where this works particularly well is in the diagnosis of rashes. The obvious visual input of a rash tends to provoke a premature pattern recognition response, i.e. I should know what that is because I can see it. By encouraging the trainee to adopt a sequential history and diagnosis and to suspend premature 'diagnostic panic', then as more data is acquired a diagnostic pattern becomes apparent.

Diagnosis directed search

If no pattern is discernible then the doctor initiates a search process. The initial symptoms and signs are analysed to produce a number of possible diagnoses (usually less than four or five). The internalised predictive values of these symptoms and signs are used to deduce the most likely diagnoses. Each diagnosis is then tested against the data until the probability diagnosis emerges. This testing is done in one of two ways: by *accumulating* and interpreting masses of data until the balance is tipped in favour of one diagnosis; or by collecting a subset of data that possesses *discriminating* qualities that allow the diagnosis to emerge. The latter process tends to be more efficient. This is the hypothetical–deductive approach used in many consultations. It requires a knowledge base, experience (which can also mislead) and ideally an idea of the predictive values of symptoms and signs (which are often not available in a useful format). Trainers can facilitate this process by providing experience, highlighting knowledge deficits and encouraging a critical approach to the acquisition of new knowledge. New knowledge should have discriminating quality. It is perhaps here that evidence-based medicine has its most appropriate application.

Systematic enquiry

Many trainers will remember being taught the 'systems enquiry' element of history taking. Many will have asked a patient presenting with OA of the knee if they had haemoptysis. Thankfully, many medical schools have realised that this is probably not a good way to learn or practice. However, *systematic scanning* is performed by doctors regularly. When a diagnosis is elusive, it can prove useful to scan for possible associated symptoms or signs that can complete the picture, i.e. with an unusual back pain enquiry about eye symptoms may elicit the history of iritis and point towards a seronegative arthritis. Most doctors develop series of scanning questions. They often start in a selected pattern (i.e. enquiry about eye, skin and bowel symptoms with arthritis) and can include opening 'screening'-type enquiry (i.e. anything wrong with your chest?) before going in a bit deeper if indicated (any cough? any blood?, etc.). Raising awareness of this process can help trainees to make better use of the battery of questions available to them.

All three of these problem-solving styles are required in general practice. The art is to use the most efficient and effective style on the day. An awareness of the styles can help both trainees and trainers to try and achieve this.

PLANNING THE TUTORIAL: A SKELETON GUIDE

This section aims to summarise the tutorial planning process combining the methods described (*see* Table 5.11).

Table 5.11 Tutorial planning structure

Task		Potential methods
Find a learning area	– knowledge	Confidence rating scales/inventories/RCGP curriculum
		MCQ, AKT or PEP tests
		Review of experience/qualifications
		RCA/feedback from staff (MSF), patients (PSQ or PUNs/DENs), note, script, referral reviews
	– skills	Observation/discussion (direct, video, COT, CbD, etc.)
		Skills lists
		Examination techniques (DOPS)
		Management (observation, feedback, experience, etc.)
	– self-awareness	Observation, discussion and feedback
	– other methods	Trainee wish list
		Specific lists (need to know, difficult list, ethics list, etc.)
		Personal construct analysis
		Review of reflective diary
		Review of problems raised by trainee (problem-based learning)

Jointly agree on learning needs	Jointly agree on aims
	Discussion and record on a tutorial planning document
	Assess learning style/personality learning style questionnaire
	Self-directed learners rating scale (SDLRS)
	Myers-Briggs type indicator
	Field dominance, hemispheric dominance, VAK preference
	Assertiveness
	Thinking style
	Discussion
Assess motivation and skill level	Motivation scale, motivation cycles
	Observation and discussion
	Skill/will matrix
Jointly agree methods	Patient-based – random or virtual case analysis/ CbD models/scripts or referral
	– video, mapping/SETGO/ Pendleton's rules/CSA type format/ COT
	– observation/models
	– joint surgeries
	– role playing
	Other methods – pictures/pre-recorded videos/ written material (guidelines, articles, questionnaire)
	– models/scripts or referral reviews/ juggling/'tips and tricks', etc.
Preparation and planning	Written on a planning form. May include (references, tutorial planning guides), 'thinking time', filling in questionnaires, collecting cases, using the internet, etc.
The tutorial event	Protected time and a suitable environment
	Appropriate resources
	'Baggage check', i.e. both trainee and trainer are ready to go
	The process – active listening
	with the trainer – appropriate questioning skills
	demonstrating: – appropriate feedback skills
	– use of a variety of educational tools
	– the encouragement of self-awareness

	– the development of problem solving skills
	– appropriate information giving behaviour
	– a sense of direction and position (i.e. not straying inappropriately off course)
	– an awareness of any appropriate emotional elements
	– enthusiasm and interest
Closing the tutorial	Reviewing aims, developing new aims
	Considering follow up sessions
	Ensuring final baggage check, i.e. are there any loose ends
	Arranging for feedback – for both parties
	Use of tutorial record form
	Discussing e-portfolio entry
	Entering clinical supervision comments/notes

This scheme can produce the same feelings in a trainer as lists of the components of a primary care consultation expected to last 10 minutes can in the new trainee. When looked at as a whole the structure simply raises to the conscious level the processes most trainers are already using to some degree. By doing this it opens up the possibility of reviewing the process and possibly improving it.

Chapter 10 will explore this area in more depth.

SUMMARY

If you fail to plan you are planning to fail. (Anon)

The art of facilitating the learning process involves juggling a number of variables. trainees have different learning styles, they think using different cognitive styles, use different problem solving styles and they have different preferences for learning environments (instructional preferences). Trainers have their own teaching styles and a tool-box of strategies to employ. Dovetailing these variables is the challenge.

Eric Jensen describes the parallels between child and adult learning (Jensen E. *Superteaching: turning points for teachers*. New York: Barron's Educational Series; 1994). Basically, he encourages more 'fun and play' with adults. He suggests the following ideal circumstances to maximise learning.

➤ Lots of play (i.e. games, tricks activities).
➤ Humour (encouraging laughter).
➤ Imagination (abstract props, interpretation).
➤ Positive support (encouragement, reinforcement, praise).
➤ Relaxation (more play, social activities).
➤ Physical activity (walks, games, etc.).
➤ Use of music and singing (tapes, videos).
➤ A rich environment – visually and physically (resources, inspiration, motivation).
➤ A good peer group.

Tutorial planning can make a huge difference to the quality of the training year. It is said there are only two real commodities in this world – time and space – and there isn't much of either! Trainers need to plan their time so they can plan their tutorials and this section may make that process a little easier.

Hemispheric dominance model (after Sperry, Gregorac, Butler and Hermann)

An appreciation of the trainee and trainer's hemispheric dominance can provide some insights that could improve the learning process. Table 5.12 can be used to inform the trainer.

Table 5.12 Hemispheric dominance model

Left dominant	Right dominant
Likes language numbers, symbols	Likes pictures/images
Verbally expressive	Demonstrative
Controlled/systematic	Open minded/random
Analytical	Creative
Prefers talking/writing	Prefers private studying
Looks for cause and effect	Experiential
Controls feelings	Free with feelings
Over-skills themselves	Tends to under-skill themselves
Reads first	Does first
Sense of time	Intuitive (often late!)
Objective	Subjective

Butler and Hermann added a further 'upper and lower' dimension to this model postulating a different role for the lower and upper cerebral hemispheres. This allowed the development of four learning styles that are described in Table 5.13.

Table 5.13

Upper left **ABSTRACT SEQUENTIAL**	Upper right **ABSTRACT RANDOM**
Parts processed better than wholes. Orderly, sequential, analytical, systematic approaches. Wants schedules and precise instruction. Prefers to work independently with a rational and intellectual approach.	Sees the whole better than the parts. Prefers abstract concepts, patterns and creative approaches. Uses non-linear, intuitive and spontaneous styles. Works independently and likes to see the whole picture.
Lower left **CONCRETE SEQUENTIAL**	Lower right **CONCRETE RANDOM**
Steady, reliable, predictable and organised. Prefers words to shapes or concepts. Likes detail and follows instruction. Prefers to work with others. Needs encouragement. Dislikes surprises. Good listeners. Likes defined problems.	Lives in the world of feelings, music, movement and relationships. Relies on doing and feeling. Sensitive to others' feelings and meanings. Restless if not doing. Likes fun. Likes others. Needs to dream, create and be challenged.

CHAPTER 6

Management and change: how do trainers use these concepts?

We trained hard, but it seemed that every time we were beginning to form up into new teams we would be re-organised. I was to learn later in life that we tend to meet any new situation by re-organising; and a wonderful method it can be for creating the illusion of progress while producing confusion, inefficiency and demoralisation. (Petronius Arbiter, Roman General, AD 66)

INTRODUCTION

The two concepts of management and change are combined in this chapter, in which we will look at tools that trainers use in this arena. If effective management is about effecting change then these two concepts belong together, and if effecting change is about understanding people (and ourselves) then this is a broad chapter!

A survey of newly vocationally trained GPs identified practice and staff management as areas of perceived deficiency in their training. This is partly explained by Laing's poem 'The Knot' (*see* Chapter 8). Many trainees 'don't know what they are supposed to know' and only find out in practice. However, the trainer does have a duty to raise awareness of this blind spot. Recently there has been an increased interest in clinicians as leaders and managers and most regions now offer leadership training courses (often university-based). It is perhaps even more important for trainers to raise the profile of this area in their trainees.

THE 'WHY' OF MANAGEMENT

A tutorial based on this question can open up awareness. The following areas could be raised for discussion.

Is the function of managing to:
➤ Educate people?
➤ Focus effort?
➤ Get the job done?
➤ Direct people because there only seems to be one solution?

➤ Be safe?
➤ Be efficient?
➤ Prevent problems?
➤ Get revenge?
➤ Prevent mistakes?
➤ Make things easier?
➤ To reward?
➤ Have control?

One trainer suggested contrasting a 'well managed' organisation with a 'badly managed' one to bring out these points. The principles of total quality management (a Japanese industrial tool where everyone is seen as a valuable contributor to a business at every level) can also be discussed. *See* at: www.businessballs. com/qualitymanagement.htm for a more detailed explanation.

THE 'HOW' OF MANAGEMENT

Personal management

Anyone who has had more than one child will realise that people seem to be fundamentally different from an early age. While it may be optimistic to expect dramatic changes in an individuals behaviour it is possible to offer practical tips.

Practical tips

An interesting distinction exists between the words 'important' and 'urgent'. Many of us spend a lot of time doing 'urgent' things. Urgency is usually defined by the needs of others, important things relate to our own needs. On occasions we need to reflect on whether the urgent task we are doing is more relevant than the important one we could be doing. This advice comes from the Irish College of GPs (time management: key ideas. In: *Handbook and Diary*. Dublin: ICGP; 1991).

➤ Work smarter not harder.
➤ Develop a sense of time.
➤ Plan ahead:
  – jobs that must be done today
  – jobs that I can delegate
  – jobs that should be done today
  – jobs that can wait
  – jobs that will never be done.
➤ Prioritise:
  – urgent, important – do it now

- non-urgent, important – assign time but do it ASAP
- urgent, unimportant – do ASAP now (perhaps!).
- non important, non urgent – only do if time permits (if at all).
➤ Identify your best times: use them productively (including for personal time). This may include quiet times to think or read, times when interruptions are unlikely, etc.
➤ Capitalise on marginal time, i.e. read when travelling, keep short jobs to hand for short time gaps.
➤ Set deadlines and finish what you start.
➤ Learn to say no.
➤ Learn to delegate.
➤ Use the telephone.
➤ Keep meetings to a minimum, keep them short and to a time plan.
➤ Learn to see problems as good – they would find you anyway!
➤ Minimise interruptions but plan for the inevitable ones.

The following advice can advice help manage the paperwork mountain.
➤ Use an in/out tray (or a virtual IT-based alternative).
➤ All mail should come via the in-tray to make prioritisation easier.
➤ Keep this tray empty – it is a mailbox only.
➤ Put as much as possible in the out tray or bin.
➤ Try not to handle the same piece of paper twice, i.e. whatever you're going to do: do it *now*.
➤ Sort large piles of paperwork on the 'three-pile system', i.e.:
  Pile 1 – I must read this
  Pile 2 – I should read this
  Pile 3 – I don't really need to read this.
  Throw pile 3 away and try and repeat the process with pile 2 until you are left with the minimum you are happy about.
➤ Consider a 'layered' filing system, i.e. a number of trays on your desk perhaps labelled:
  Tray 1 – do today
  Tray 2 – do this week
  Tray 3 – do sometime
  Tray 4 – projects.
  Aim to keep Tray 1 clear. Review the second daily and the third when you have time. If any paperwork remains unactioned for more than a week reconsider if it should be there at all.
➤ Diary use: use your diary (written, electronic or e-portfolio) to record anything you would like to remember, but might forget – not just appointments but patients you are particularly worried about or questions

that occur to you (Could I learn to excise a chalazion? How often do other people do U&Es in patients on ACEIs?) If you get into this habit and review your diary on a daily basis then your mind does not carry these thoughts and worries around all day and they are not lost forever. If you get to the entry in the diary and feel unmoved to action then put a line through the entry and move on. It also tends to be a lot tidier that 20 post-its stuck on your desk!

Problem-solving methods

A number of approaches to problem analysis and ways of producing change were mentioned by trainers. These vary from the short acronym to the in-depth psychoanalytical tool. Trainers will have to consider the depth of approach the particular trainee and particular problem require.

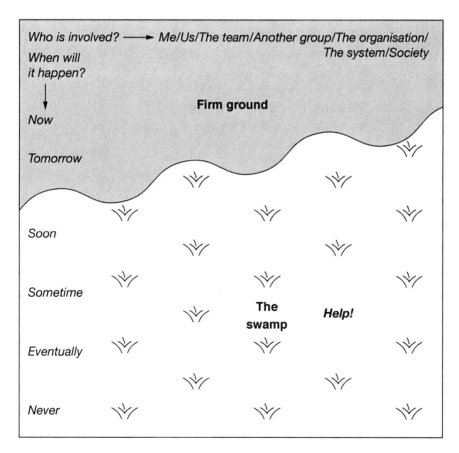

Figure 6.1: Management: spheres of influence.

Action planning

This is a three-step process to encourage realistic goals for change.

Step 1:   Use Figure 6.1 to make sure you are not in the 'swamp', i.e. the change you hope to achieve is within your sphere of influence.

Step 2:   Be specific – i.e. define what you want to achieve and how to achieve it.

Step 3:   Ask WHY? WHO? WHEN? WHERE? HOW? WHAT?

GROW, SMART and FRAME

A number of short acronyms exist to help the trainer structure short interactions where change is sought by the learner. three of these are described below.

GROW

This technique is really designed for the 15–30-minute interaction with a learner to help them find a way forward with a problem.

G – goals –   What would you like to achieve in this session?

What needs to happen for you to achieve your aim?

Will this be of real value to you?

Is it a realistic aim?

R – reality –   What is happening now? How often? When does it happen?

Is this an accurate assessment?

What effect does this have?

What other factors are relevant?

Who else is involved? What is their perception?

What have you tried so far? (encouraging self-assessment)

O – options –   What can you do? (all options)

Who or what could help?

Would you like suggestions?

Which options interest you most Why?

What are the pros and cons here?

Rate the options 1–10 on practicality.

Would you like to choose one option now?

W – wrap up –   What are the next steps?

When will you take them?

What might hinder your plans?

What support do you need? How and when will you get it?

How will you know you have achieved your goals?

FRAME

This can be a useful aide-memoir for planning educational objectives for both learners and trainers.

F –   few –   set one or only a few goals

R –   realistic –   make the goals achievable

A – agreed –   if the process involves others enlist their support and agreement

M – measurable – make sure you will know when the goal is achieved

E – explicit –   try to exclude hidden agendas and keep the process open.

SMART

This is very similar to the FRAME technique. It stresses relevance and timing which may be more appropriate for some trainees.

S – specific –   set a specific objective

M – measurable – make it measurable

A – attainable –   make it attainable

R – relevant –   make it relevant

T – timed –   time frame the process.

Navigation

This is a series of three questions to ask when you set off on the 'journey' of change. Each question contains a number of secondary elements.

1 Where am I/we now? How did we get here? Did the experience teach us anything?
2 Where do I/we want to be? What are our real priorities and how do they fit with this goal?
   Why do we want to go there? Who is involved?
3 How am I/are we going to get there? What will help us? What will hinder us? What routes are possible? With what implications?
   How will we know we've arrived? (Will we arrive or overshoot?)

POSSEER exercise

This is an exercise in assessing the opportunity for change and helping a person to identify a path forward. You work through the ill-defined problem or goal using the acronym.

P – positive –   make sure the goal is stated on positive terms, i.e. 'I'm always late' becomes 'I want to be on time'.

O – owned –   define what is in the person's power to achieve, i.e. if you are always late because there is no public transport then you can't catch an earlier bus.

S – specific –   define the how, what, where, when and who.

S – size –   make it a balance between possibility and challenge, i.e. not too small or too big.

E – evidence –   how will it be evident the change has occurred? This needs to be explicit.

E – ecology –   how will the change fit into the persons wider existence?

R – resources – are the tools for the job available?

The aim is to leave the person feeling that the goal is achievable in a practical sense and therefore motivate them to go for it. The facilitator should be able to get an 'acceptance set' (*see* Chapter 7 in response to the question 'are you going to do that then?' at the end of the exercise).

Cognitive therapy

The roots of cognitive therapy probably lie in the Socratic style of teaching. Socrates is purported to have helped an uneducated slave prove Pythagoras' theorem *simply* by asking questions. He achieved this by encouraging the learner to critically examine their own observations, thoughts, feelings and experiences and to use new insights to build self-constructed concepts on secure foundations. Easy! The cognitive therapy model aims to make this process accessible to the rest of us. For example let's assume a trainee's surgeries always run very late: a jointly developed analysis of the situation may be as shown in Figure 6.2.

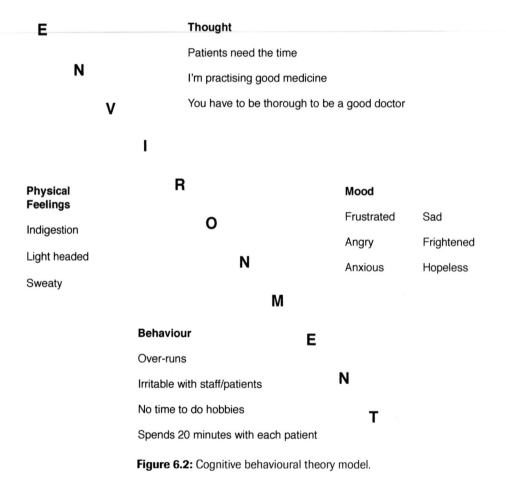

E   **Thought**

N

Patients need the time

I'm practising good medicine

V

You have to be thorough to be a good doctor

I

R

Physical Feelings   **Mood**

Indigestion   **O**   Frustrated   Sad

Light headed   Angry   Frightened

N

Sweaty   Anxious   Hopeless

M

Behaviour   **E**

Over-runs

Irritable with staff/patients   **N**

No time to do hobbies

T

Spends 20 minutes with each patient

Figure 6.2: Cognitive behavioural theory model.

The behaviours, moods, thoughts and physical feelings are analysed and placed on the framework as shown above. The trainer facilitates this process by bringing out unconscious or hidden elements. The framework can then be used to develop strategies for change which can range from simple symptom management (relaxation techniques) to behavioural change (book patients at 20-minute intervals for now and have some sessions on consultation skills) and even to looking at value systems (What is 'good' medicine? Who has first call on your time?). It is not suggested that every problem needs this in-depth approach although it does seem a useful way to identify the causes, effects and possible solution areas when change is necessary.

Logical levels exercise

There are at least two versions of this exercise that can be done with pen and paper (perhaps for the theorist) or physically 'hopping' on a series of cards (for the activist). It asserts that a problem or perceived need for change can be looked at on a number of levels.

Level 1   What is the problem?
Level 2   What do I feel about the problem?
Level 3   What do I think about the problem?
Level 4   What values do I have around this issue?
Level 5   What beliefs underpin my values?

The trainee is taken through this process by considering a number of questions – these can be written on cards and placed on the floor. The trainee hops from one question to the next describing their responses at each station.

Q1   Where are you? (scene setting)
Q2   What is the problem area for change? (clarifying goal)
Q3   How do you feel about this? (feelings)
Q4   What are you thinking about this? (thoughts)
Q5   What do these thoughts mean? (interpretation)
Q6   Why do you believe they mean this? (values)
Q7   Who are you?   (personal comfort/role)
Q8   Are you comfortable with your beliefs? (beliefs)
Q9   Is change still necessary? (check problem still real)
Q10   Name a specific change you can make? (identify change)

Enough insight or need for change may develop at any question level and the process can stop at this point. If the trainee completes the process they can run back through the questions (starting at Q1 imagining the change has occurred). This can help check that the proposed change feels appropriate.

The second approach suggests a number of stations – each analysed to try to develop insight into why the desired change is a problem.

1	Place	– is the physical environment the issue?
2	Behaviour	– is the desired behaviour possible?
3	Capability	– do I have the necessary skills?
4	Beliefs	– do I believe this outcome is desirable?
5	Values	– do I value this outcome personally?
6	Identity	– does the desired outcome fit with my view of myself?
7	Spirituality	– does this outcome fit with my concepts of humanity?

A simpler model can also be useful (*see* Figure 6.3).

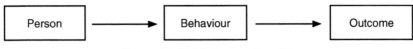

Figure 6.3 NLP behavioural model.

In other words, is the 'block' for change situated in the person, the behaviour required or is it the outcome that is the problem?

Many of these concepts come from euro-linguistic Programming: *see* the resources section for further details or visit www.businessballs.com/nlpneurolinguisticprogramming.htm

Chaos theory

Complexity and chaos theory have evolved as a major alternative to the analytical/logico-deductive approach to change and can offer insights into change in complex systems (i.e. general practice, patients and medicine in general!). This is a complex area but the major messages are that in-depth analysis of complex situations will often not lead to constructive outcomes but an awareness of emergent patterns (attractors), the recognition of a minimum number of required conditions linked to a vision of direction and a sensitivity to evolving change will allow the situation to develop a satisfactory outcome. For an excellent and quite brief description of the concepts involved, visit www.resources.scalingtheheights.com/the_edge_of_chaos.htm

It is not clear how trainers use this in practice but the training process and general practice are definitely chaotic and awareness of this theory may help trainees who adopt a rather rigid or over-analytical approach.

SWOT analysis

The SWOT technique describes a tool designed to facilitate the analysis of a situation where no clear cut solution or way forward exists. The situation is analysed under the four headings.

S   trengths

W eaknesses

O   pportunities

T   hreats

The process illustrates the links between threats and opportunities, strengths and weaknesses and encourages all parties to contribute to an overall picture. Hopefully, a more balanced decision emerges.

Narrative theory

Narrative theory in medicine is another relatively new concept – it seems to provide a focus for many of the ideas that have been around for a number of years. Humans have told stories as a way of understanding their existence since prehistoric times and doctors can learn empathic skills and broaden their own understanding by adopting a narrative-based stance. The use of stories ('cases') has been the backbone of medical education since Hippocrates and an understanding of how and why we tell our stories can broaden the educational experience.

What does this mean for trainers? A number of suggestions were made.

➤ The use of film and book resources can be a way to develop trainees empathic skills (*see* the resources section).

➤ Painting a picture or writing a poem (*see* the advice sheet in the CD-ROM) can be a good way of exploring a problem or a consultation.

➤ Exploring 'family scripts' can offer insights that broaden our understanding – these are the 'programmes' we received in our upbringing, i.e. 'hard work is good', 'duty is of paramount importance', 'mothers should look after children' – making them explicit can be an revealing exercise!

➤ The deliberate search for metaphor (our own and the patient's) can deepen our understanding of the patients 'mind map' – *see* at: www. resources.scalingtheheights.com/the_edge_of_chaos.htm

➤ The concept of 'clean language' can be a useful way of exploring how we use our verbal skills – *see* the article at: www.cleanlanguage.co.uk/articles/ articles/30/1/Tangled-Spaghetti-in-My-Head-Making-use-of-metaphor/ Page1.html

There are now whole medical school courses based on this concept!

Some thoughts on change

Why is change so difficult to achieve sometimes and so automatic at others? Three areas shed some light on this question.

A – Habits: we are creatures of habit and once we have developed a pattern of behaviour we derive security from this and resist losing it.

B – Externalisations: if we perceive that an external force has control we are often slow to recognise our own control (i.e. the locus of control theory).

C – Self-disciplines: even if we perceive the need for change it requires motivation and drive to achieve it.

The 'four fears' often act as additional blocks to change:
1 fear of failure
2 fear of change (the 'devil I know' syndrome)
3 fear of self-confrontation/self-exposure
4 fear of success.

These ideas can be helpful in the analysis of difficult situations.

The 'ZPD' – Zone of Proximal Development (Vygotsky)

This is a useful concept for trainers. Vygotsky suggested educators need to find the zone just beyond where the learner is currently and then build a 'scaffold' to encourage the learner to explore. This is what trainers do all the time I hear you say!

Motivation

Many trainers feel that high motivation is one of the key elements of successful training. Maslow's scale (with Neighbour's modification) and Glasser's table provide some insights in this area (*see* introduction in Chapter 2). The rank ordering scale (*see* at: www.radcliffepublishing.com/gptrainershandbook) is a practical tool to help analyse driving forces. What other ways do trainers use to look at the problem of motivation? The two cycles of demotivation are shown in Figures 6.4 and 6.5.

If the trainee is within the negative cycle of demotivation the trainer can highlight the problem and work on confidence building, i.e. jointly select an area where good performance can be anticipated (everyone has some good

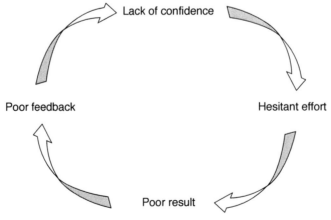

Figure 6.4: Negative cycle of demotivation.

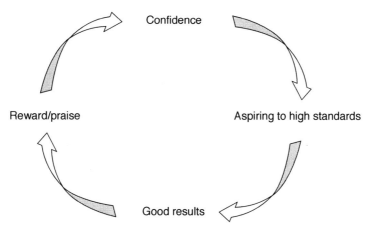

Figure 6.5: Positive cycle of demotivation.

potential skills), construct a plan and ensure plenty of feedback. If the trainee is in the positive cycle of demotivation it is usually a lack of reward or praise that is the problem. Doctors are notoriously poor at providing positive feedback. A simple 'well done' or acknowledgement of patient satisfaction can have an enormous effect.

In Motivation to learn. *British Journal of General Practice.* 1998; 48: 1429–32. Miller *et al.* looked specifically at motivation to learn in GPs. They propose a developmental view of learning motivations. A simplification of this approach is summarised in Table 6.1.

Table 6.1 Developmental view of motivation to learn in GPs

Stages	INNATE	EARLY LEARNING	SOCIALISATION	PROFESSIONALISATION	INDEPENDENCE
Motivators	Curiosity Altruism	Inventive Role models	Peer pressure	Professional values Reputation Security Job satisfaction	Pragmatism
Type of learner	Global unfocussed	Superficial	Deep	Strategic	Tactical

This model encourages us to accept that different motivators are at work in different learners. It can help us to appreciate and perhaps harness the trainee's motivators and encourages the concept of developing their motivations by trying to move the learner towards the right of the scale above. This involves stimulating individual development perhaps by raising awareness of professional values and the breadth of general practice. Providing appropriate role models is also highlighted.

The motivating skills questionnaire can provide trainers with some insight into their own motivating skills. The questionnaire is designed to assess a person's managerial skill in motivating others. It can act as an interesting stimulus to discussion in this area. *See* www.radcliffepublishing.com/gptrainershandbook

Two more brief motivation concepts can also have uses in understanding our trainees.

1   Is the motivation 'head' or 'heart'? i.e. logical or emotive – often the former is used as on overlay when the latter is at work!
2   Are the learners motivated *toward* or *away from*? Are they forward or backward focused? Would reinforcing either of these perspectives affect motivation?

THE 'WHAT' OF MANAGEMENT

In response to the comments of many newly vocationally trained GPs (who express anxieties about their training in this area), some trainers use a list of management areas for the trainee to consider. The list aims to open the trainees' eyes to the scope of the management role to enable them to define their own learning objectives. A sample list is shown in the appendix to this chapter (*see also* www.radcliffepublishing.com/gptrainershandbook). The appendix also contains an in-depth look at the insurance element of running a practice. This can be a useful tool for discussion and tend to open a trainee's perspective of practice management.

Teams

The need to function within a team is an essential element of modern general practice. Trainees need to be suitably equipped to achieve this. The following sections offer resources to stimulate thought in this area.

Many trainers find Belbin's team style inventory useful in this contest. The *Self perception inventory* is based on a questionnaire and allocates a score reflecting your team role strengths. The categories are as follows.

➤ Chairperson – director.
➤ Company worker – practical and efficient.
➤ Completer finisher – task orientated driving force.
➤ Monitor evaluator – analytical and checking.
➤ Resource investigator – looks externally for resources.
➤ Team worker – supportive.
➤ Shaper – looks at objectives and outcome.
➤ Plant – looks for novel solutions.

At the assessment level it gives the trainer an insight into the trainees normal team behaviour and raises awareness of team functions. See the link at: www.belbin.com

Characteristics of effective teams

This is a list of the ideal team components for discussion.

➤ **Vision and common purpose**

The team members know why the team exists. They have clear objectives and a shared vision. They focus on results and are good at setting priorities and making decisions.

➤ **Communication**

This is vital, open and honest. Feedback is valued and conflict resolved. Team members listen, say what they think and respect others' views. Team members are able to challenge each other with no hidden agendas.

➤ **Trust and respect**

All team members are valued and supported as valid contributors to the whole performance.

➤ **Shared leadership**

Leadership is not based on status or position. The formal leader is a coach and mentor. The appropriate leader(s) emerges and all team members take responsibility for decisions. When necessary a leader to take quick decisions emerges. Team members are empowered to take part in decision-making where appropriate.

➤ **Procedural**

The team develops policies and rules designed to help achieve goals. The team is efficient at gathering information, mustering resources, organising and evaluating. Creativity, innovation and good risk assessment are all valued.

➤ **Flexibility and adaptability**

The team sees change as an opportunity more than a threat. The team is constantly looking to improve processes and tends to delegate this to appropriate members.

➤ **Team roles**

The team recognises different strengths in different members and sees this as a resource to use and learn from. The team looks for gaps in its function and seeks to remedy these by training, recruitment or outside resource use.

➤ **Learning**

The team takes measured risks and learns from mistakes. There is an expectation of individual growth and an encouragement of questions. They expect learning opportunities in all situations. Actions are considered, agreed and evaluated. New learning produces appropriate change.

Behaviours seen in effective teams

This list can look superficially similar to the one above, but is looking at the same elements from a behavioural point of view. This allows more analysis of where problems might lie and also points towards solutions. It has a more pragmatic feel to it than the more theoretical list of ideals above.

➤ **Clear goals**

Team roles are clarified (job descriptions, titles, areas of responsibility).
Acceptable differences are defined (codes of conduct, disciplinary codes, dress codes, contracts).
Values are discussed and consensus reached (meeting forums, mission statements).

➤ **Support and trust**

Feelings are recognised and dealt with (feedback systems, support networks).
People display empathy, respect and are genuine (no cliques, no jealousies, people chose to spend time and talk together at and across all levels of the organisation).
Individual worries are shared in a supportive manner.

➤ **Communication**

Honest feedback is given sensitively (positive and negative) to everyone (appraisals, reward systems).
People communicate well person to person.

➤ **Conflict**

Conflicts are seen as inevitable and sources of growth.
Conflicts are dealt with rapidly.
All parties are encouraged to be assertive.
Discussions are 'solution-based' and people are not blamed.
Attempts are made to minimise areas of conflict.

➤ **Procedures**

There are clear procedures that are helpful (protocols, policies).
Delegation is explicit and empowering.
Meetings are actively managed (agendas, times, minutes, actions).

➤ **Leadership**

The leadership is constructive and uses the strengths of the team.

➤ **Evaluation**

The team reviews its progress (audits, reports, use of data).
This process is focused on producing a better result.

➤ **Individual development**

The team aims to promote improvement in the performance of all members (appraisals, training, courses, promotion).

➤ **Perspective**

The team looks both inwards and outwards to build relationships (other commitments, links to other bodies, use of outside resources).

Assertiveness

Assertiveness is seen as one of the important elements of the effective team member. Many individuals' assertiveness skills are either non-existent or linked to an aggressive approach. This not only reduces there effectiveness but produces collateral damage as it offends others or leaves them frustrated. *See* www. radcliffepublishing.com/gptrainershandbook for the assertion rights questionnaire. This enables the trainer to look at this emotive area through the 'third party' of the questionnaire. In practice this tends to make the exercise less threatening. The result produces a combination of the 'OK' and 'NOT OK' scenarios, shown in Box 6.1.

BOX 6.1

I'M OK, YOU'RE OK – ASSERTIVE BEHAVIOUR – WIN/WIN
We value each other and ourselves, listen to each other and share our thoughts and feelings honestly.

I'M NOT OK, YOU'RE OK – PASSIVE BEHAVIOUR – LOSE/WIN
I think you embody what I am not and although I respect you I don't think you really want to hear what I have to say. It's easier to keep quiet and do want you want me to because I want you to like me and I don't feel equal to you.

I'M OK, YOU'RE NOT OK – AGGRESSIVE BEHAVIOUR – WIN/LOSE
I think I know better and are more important than you. I may interrupt and ignore you. I don't really need to make much effort to let you have what you're entitled to.

I'M NOT OK, YOU'RE NOT OK – INDIRECT AGGRESSION – LOSE/ LOSE
I don't have much faith in you, or myself. I feel at war with you but would not tell you that. I have little self-respect so I avoid issues, preferring to use insincere praise and flattery to try and get my way. I will try and undermine you behind your back.

Assertiveness 'bill of rights'

This is a simple list of individual rights. A discussion or even a rank ordering of this list can be a useful tool for identifying values and attitudes in this area. trainers have found this useful when they have identified potential problems in trainees:

➤ to be treated with respect as a capable and equal human being
➤ to have and express my own feelings, values and opinions without having to justify or apologise for them

➤ to be listened to seriously
➤ to set my own priorities and state my own needs and be myself – not what others want or expect me to be
➤ to say yes or no for myself without guilt
➤ to have the right to make mistakes and to change my mind sometimes
➤ to ask for what I want accepting that I may not always get it
➤ to say I don't understand
➤ to choose not to be assertive.

Assertiveness training

These simple techniques can be offered to the trainee with problems.
1 Ownership – use 'I' statements, i.e. 'I think'; 'I want'.
2 Don't ramble – try to state your words concisely and clearly.
3 Ask questions – ask open questions to establish other peoples' opinions, i.e. I'm not sure about this.
4 Listen – learn to actively listen at all times.
5 Involvement – try to reduce the emotional content in both yourself and others when being assertive, i.e. 'I'm not trying to make you angry'; 'I'm sorry if this upsets you but we do need to sort it out'.
6 Say what you want.
7 Set limits – so you can't be manipulated.
8 'Broken record' technique – keep repeating your view if you are feeling ignored.

Leadership

> The true leader is always led. (Jung)

Many people would suggest that an awareness of leadership skills is essential for the GP. Recently, there has been a major initiative to provide leadership training for clinicians in recognition of the importance of this area and both trainers and trainees may benefit by enrolling on these schemes.

The following lists can provide a basis for discussion.
1 Questions
   ➤ Name four leaders – Were they successful? What skills did they possess? (Try it on Hitler and Churchill or politicians or sportsmen.)
   ➤ Think of someone you have had personal contact with as a leader? Why were you impressed?
   ➤ What are the skills the perfect leader would have?
   ➤ How does someone acquire these skills?
   ➤ Where have you seen effective/less effective leadership in the practice?

2   Good leadership is characterised by:
   ➤ continuity
   ➤ willingness to invest time
   ➤ a vision of the goal
   ➤ ability to motivate others
   ➤ a belief in the goal
   ➤ an overall perception of the situation
   ➤ energy and enthusiasm
   ➤ ability to see and get the best from others.
3   The functions of a leader include:
   ➤ establishing, communicating and clarifying goals
   ➤ motivating
   ➤ establishing processes
   ➤ setting standards
   ➤ acting as a role model (*see* Table 6.3)
   ➤ encouraging and rewarding
   ➤ monitoring and evaluating
   ➤ maximising resource efficiency
   ➤ providing feedback
   ➤ highlighting foreseeable problems.

Delegation

Effective management has been defined as 'performing tasks through others'. If this is true then delegation is a core skill for general practitioners. This section looks at the use of delegation as a teaching tool and describes some thoughts on delegation that may help in tutorial design.

Delegation as a teaching tool – the skill/will matrix

Trainers need to know how to delegate, when to delegate and how to facilitate the development of delegation skills in learners. Delegation is sometimes desirable but not advisable. The skill/will matrix is an interesting way of analysing this situation. Table 6.2 illustrates this technique. The trainer must form an opinion of the trainee's skill level and motivation for a particular aspect of training. The matrix then suggests appropriate training techniques to improve the probability that learning will occur.

The term 'coaching' is defined in Chapter 5. Directive coaching commits the trainer to two tasks: first, the provision of a safe, structured and controlled environment for learning; and, secondly, the duty to analyse and stimulate motivation. Delegative coaching involves a more hands-off approach to the high achiever whilst remaining available for feedback and consultation. The aim is to develop the learner's skills and stimulate their motivation to allow

Table 6.2 Skill/will matrix

	High skill	*Deficient skill*
High will	*Peak performer*	*Enthusiastic beginner*
Method	Delegative coaching	Supervisory coaching
	Help to set objectives (not methods)	Provide structure
	Praise (not ignore)	Control and supervise closely
	Devolve decision-making	Use informative questions
	Use interpretative questions	Praise/listen and facilitate
	Increase awareness of potential	Safety net to allow mistakes – be slow to chide
Low will	*Reluctant contributor*	*Disillusioned learner*
Method	Excite/motivate/supportive coaching	Directive coaching
	Analyse motivation	Look at motivation
	Provide stimulation	Look at ability
	Look for personal problems	Clear communication lines
	Praise, listen and facilitate	Develop a path forwards
		Provide positive feedback opportunities (i.e. play to strengths)
		Control, supervise and structure

the delegative style. This matrix has the potential to help trainers and trainees design appropriate educational experiences.

Teaching delegation skills

Many trainees have to adapt to the process of delegation in the practice with little awareness of the principles. The following points may help open this area up in a tutorial.

What are the purposes of delegation?
➤ to deal with the task effectively *and* efficiently
➤ to ensure optimum use of capacity
➤ to free up the delegator to allow them to use time for more important tasks
➤ to stimulate staff and increase their competencies
➤ to create an atmosphere of achievement and responsibility
➤ sometimes to increase financial rewards.

It should *not*:
➤ create a feeling of dumping on staff
➤ lower standards
➤ overload staff.

Why don't people delegate more? A number of possible reasons are listed below. Sometimes it is simply that we are 'intimidated by talent' as one manager put it.

➤ It upsets one's ego (no-one else can do it, can they?).
➤ Anxiety about mistakes (I'm the only one who doesn't make mistakes).
➤ Anxiety about the process (my way is the only way).
➤ Fear of loss of control (I'm the boss).
➤ Desire for perfection (no-one else will do it as well as I can).
➤ Lack of confidence in others (they are all useless).
➤ False sense of efficiency (I can do everything anyway).

So what about the principles of good delegation? Table 6.3 shows the 'Nine-point guide to perfect delegation'. Point 5 involves the completed staffwork concept. This was a tool described by Napoleon Bonaparte. If there was a problem in the army and his General asked for a solution then he was dismissed. If the General had analysed the situation and developed the options he could stay, i.e. the delegator should expect to advise and not sort things out themselves.

Table 6.3 The nine-point guide to perfect delegation

1	Select the right person
2	Give them explicit instructions
3	Provide them with the tools for the job
4	Assign a task and an outcome (but not exactly how to do it)
5	Use the completed staffwork system
6	Don't attach strings (i.e. allow them to think and develop)
7	Resist upward delegation (i.e. 'How did you want me to do this?')
8	Agree a deadline
9	Follow through (i.e. feedback and monitor)

When you delegate to someone make sure you give them the responsibility that goes with the task, the authority to do it and the accountability for the result.

Where possible it is helpful to delegate an area of management to the trainee. Examples have included a role in the winter flu vaccination campaign, the purchase of a piece of equipment, the writing and implementation of a new policy, etc. An audit project has potential in this area.

The five delegation zones.

Zone 1 – Tasks that *cannot* be delegated.
Zone 2 – Tasks which the delegator should deal with. These should only really be delegated if professionally acceptable and under extreme time pressure or if the delegation is more in the form of assistance, i.e. the responsibility remains with the delegator.

Zone 3 – Tasks that *could* be delegated. The delegator has the most appropriate skills but other staff could do this with support and training.

Zone 4 – Tasks that *should* be delegated. Other staff have the skills to do this already.

Zone 5 – Tasks that *must* be delegated. These are the tasks that the delegator may have process knowledge of but does not possess the skills to perform.

It can be an interesting exercise to go through a surgery looking at which zone the various tasks completed fall into. This can be particularly relevant to the trainee who runs very late or fails to use the PHCT effectively.

Other points to note

Table 6.4 illustrates the relationship in the managerial environment between performance and satisfaction. This has implications for the training environment. Achieving a balance between the two elements of performance pressure and need for satisfaction can be difficult. We must try and aim to work in the integrative arena.

Table 6.4 Performance and satisfaction in the working/learning environment

		Emphasis on performance	
		LOW	HIGH
Emphasis on	LOW	INDULGING	IMPOSING
satisfaction	HIGH	IGNORING	INTEGRATING

Equation of task performance

If the trainer or trainee are armchair mathematicians or have strong theorist tendencies then they may find Maier and Lawler's formulae food for thought (*see* Box 6.2).

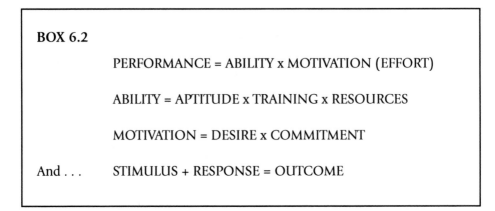

BOX 6.2

PERFORMANCE = ABILITY x MOTIVATION (EFFORT)

ABILITY = APTITUDE x TRAINING x RESOURCES

MOTIVATION = DESIRE x COMMITMENT

And . . .   STIMULUS + RESPONSE = OUTCOME

SUMMARY

Postgraduate training is all about adult education. The responsibility for learning and changing lie with the trainee. It may be helpful to look at the principles of the adult learning process and these are shown in Table 6.5.

Table 6.5 Principles of adult learning

The most effective learning occurs when:
➤ a good learner/facilitator (not teacher!) relationship exists
➤ adults select their own learning experiences (self-directed)
➤ there is an environment where new skills can be practised readily
➤ their past experience/learning is taken into account
➤ their learning styles are taken into account
➤ there are opportunities for the learner to pass on their own wisdom
➤ there is a non-threatening environment
➤ there is a good available standard they can use to assess themselves by
➤ they can assess their own progress towards personal goals.

Adult learners bring expectations, intentions, life skills and real-life demands to the learning environment and trainers need to recognise these. Trainers need to keep the learning process focused on its relevant context, i.e. clinical teaching should involve clinical material and similarly management teaching should involve management material. This is emphasised because much of this section has described techniques that seem a little distant from the real world. They must be seen as complementary techniques or even diagnostic techniques. The bulk of management training should involve placing the trainee in management scenarios for experiential learning. Many of the techniques described increase the potential for learning and change.

THE 'WHAT' OF MANAGEMENT

In-depth insurance analysis

This is an in-depth pneumonic to use as a tool to raise awareness of the complexity of practice management by looking at one area – the insurance aspects of practice.

I	Insure in everyone's sight	Impossible to self-insure
	If it can go wrong it will	Insure with professionals
	Insurance products do change	Insist on regular reviews/re-quotes
	Instigate actions to reduce risk	Insist premiums are itemised
N	Never fail to report incidents	Never fail to disclose
	Never underinsure	New circumstances must be notified
	Never underestimate exposure	Never be complacent
S	Sleep at night	Security of policies and documents
	Stage payments	Spouse protection
	Staff risks – fraud/indemnity	Sessional staff cover
	Stamp duties – hidden charges	Structure of practice can affect cover
	Special areas – product liability	
U	Use a valuer for building insurance	Use an insurance broker
	Unforced entry may not be covered under statutory obligations – public liability	
R	Read the policy	Risk assessment – do one
	Report claims promptly in writing	Review coverage regularly
	Report events	Rental properties are special considerations
E	Expect explanation of policy	Ensure you know the exclusions
	External party exposure	Expect only one insurer to pay out
	Exposure professionally	Extensions to policies
	Excess amounts	Earnings – loss of

Major areas to cover

➤ Buildings and fixtures.
➤ Contents.
➤ Computers – including data reinstatement.
➤ Loss of earnings.
➤ House and contents.
➤ Loss of life.
➤ Motor vehicles.
➤ Public liability.
➤ Product liability.

➤ Professional liability.
➤ Staff liability.
➤ Special events.
➤ Machinery breakdown.

The 'what' of management list

Practice organisation

This document is designed to raise an awareness of practice management in trainees. You should have a passing acquaintance with the following documents.

➤ Types of contract (GMS, PMS, PMS plus, confederations, QOF).
➤ Terms and conditions of employment.
➤ A practice management textbook – *see* Chapter 8.

The following list is intended as a template to help you gather the relevant information.

STAFFING

➤ 'Hiring and firing', i.e. job descriptions/contracts/legal requirements and employment law/disciplinary procedures/pay and tax/staff acquisition/ training and qualifications/assessment and development/reimbursements/ posts in practice/human resources issues/health and safety issues/equal opportunities issues.

PARTNERSHIP

➤ Sorts of jobs available (locum/assistant/salaried/part-time/retainer/share, etc.).
➤ Partnership agreements.
➤ Selection processes.
➤ Common pitfalls/survival techniques.
➤ Single-handed posts.
➤ Working as a locum.

FINANCES

➤ Money in: Health Authority/private work/outside commitments/ entrepreneurial.
➤ Money out.
➤ Reimbursements.
➤ Personal aspects: salary/tax/accountancy/, etc.
➤ Capital costs – buildings/equipment/cost rent scheme.
➤ Insurance.

DRUGS

➤ Dispensing/personally administered items.

PACT

➤ Incentive schemes.

PRIMARY CARE TRUSTS
➤ Principles.
➤ Main practical elements, i.e. budget setting/budget components/contracts/ savings/QOF/inspections/appraisal.
➤ Governance.
➤ Alternative systems.

ADMINISTRATION
➤ Computing: potential uses/links/PCT/targets/data manipulation, etc.
➤ Paperwork: forms/returns/in-house systems/medical record systems.

ADVERTISEMENT
➤ 'Selling' the practice/viability and growth.
➤ Relationship with outside agencies/reps/, etc.
➤ Relationship with Health Authority/hospitals/LMC/local trusts, etc.

IT
➤ Computers in the surgery/decision support systems/patient education.
➤ Computers in management.
➤ External links (HA/hospitals/internet/other).

OTHER
➤ (Add any more that occur to you).

CHAPTER 7

The consultation: how do trainers teach consultation skills?

Communication is the most important tool the physician can possess.
Learn to respect it and use it wisely. (Meador)

INTRODUCTION

Most trainers feel that the development of a trainee's interest in consultation skills is central to the GP training year. Raising the trainee's awareness of the communication dynamics at work in the consultation, and to see them developing these skills is for most of us a tremendously rewarding experience.

This chapter describes the techniques trainers use to teach consultation skills. These methods can be grouped into those involving patients or patient scenarios (video, role play or joint consultations) and those using other resources. The last element of this section looks at the assessment of consulting skills.

PATIENT CONTACT-RELATED METHODS

Use of video

It is almost unanimous amongst trainers that video is one of the most effective ways to teach and explore consultation skills. It is also almost unanimous that trainees will often suffer from 'video allergy'. How can this be avoided?

1 Introduce video early – probably within the first two weeks.
2 Show a video of your own surgery.
3 Have a set video surgery, e.g. once a week to get in the habit.
4 Make sure reception are involved as they will need to inform patients and obtain their consent.
5 Regularly review videos; if you have concerns over a trainee's consultation skills, ask to see a whole surgery as opposed to those that have been 'cherry picked' by the trainee.

Not surprisingly, video was the most common tool used. But how is it used? A number of strategies were mentioned.

CONSULTATION MAPPING

(*See* www.radcliffepublishing.com/gptrainershandbook) This is a process of categorising what is happening in the consultation. It seems to assume the consultation should progress through a sequence of events to produce a satisfactory outcome. Most trainers feel that this is a questionable assumption. (Notice the use of the word 'assume': it makes an ASS out of U and ME!) However, it can be a helpful starting point. Initially, it may give the trainee a form of security in being able to define a structure for the consultation. It is also helpful for those trainees who seem to struggle with the structure of the consultation and it does cover all the major elements one would hope to see.

CONSULTATION MODELLING

Some trainers feel consultation models are about as much use in teaching consultation skills as airfix models are if you want to fly! However, many would not share that view. The recurring criticism from trainees tends to be 'but this is just a way of describing what is happening anyway'. Therefore, introducing the models as 'cold theory' is quite a challenge. It is often more effective to introduce them at opportune times such as reflecting on a dysfunctional consultation. A good description of the models is available from many sources and the References section contains the relevant details. The different models have different perspectives that lend themselves to teaching consultation skills in different areas of need. The following is a brief description of each.

RCGP model

This simply asks the doctor to look beyond the organic and include the psychosocial elements of presentations and ill health – physical, psychological and social – encouraging the doctor to extend his thinking into these dimensions with each presentation.

Stott and Davies's 1979 Model

This is very task orientated. Many trainers feel a fifth task (are there any administrative elements to this consultation?) should be added to the four original ones. This can be a useful model to expand the trainee's outlook, particularly into the realms of prevention. It has no overtly psychodynamic elements and many trainers felt this was a major drawback.
➤ Management of presenting problems.
➤ Modification of help seeking behaviour.
➤ Management of continuing problems.
➤ Opportunistic health promotion (administrative element).

It can also illustrate that we were interested in health prevention even before it was worth five QOF points.

Byrne and Long's 1976 model

This is a mechanistic model that was derived from the analysis of many consultations. Their book is fairly short and has some interesting comments on dysfunctional consultations and attempts to change doctor behaviour.

Most trainers felt the model had limited application in this area.

Phase 1   The doctor establishes a relationship with the patient.

Phase 2   The doctor attempts to discover the reason for the consultation.

Phase 3   The doctor conducts a verbal and/or physical examination.

Phase 4   The doctor, or the doctor and patient, or the patient consider the problem.

Phase 5   The doctor, and occasionally the patient, discuss management.

Phase 6   The consultation is terminated.

Pendleton *et al*.'s 1984 model

This combines a structural element with a psychodynamic element and is the basis of many of the consultation maps around (*see* Table 7.1).

Tate P. *The Doctor's Communication Handbook.* 2nd ed. Oxford: Radcliffe Medical Press; 1998 is considered essential reading by many trainers and is undoubtedly useful in teaching consultation skills. Many trainers particularly mentioned Pendleton's rules, described in the book as a method of giving feedback in the video-based tutorial. These will be described later in this chapter.

Table 7.1

➤ Define the reason for attendance:	– nature and history of problems
	– their aetiology
	– the patient's ideas/concerns/ expectations
	– the effects of the problem.
➤ Consider other problems:	– continuing problems
	– at risk factors.
➤ Choose an appropriate action for each problem with the patient.	
➤ Achieve an understanding with the patient.	
➤ Involve the patient in the management plan with some responsibility for it.	
➤ To use time and resources appropriately.	
➤ To establish/maintain the appropriate relationship with the patient.	

Helman's 1984 model

This is an anthropological model and helps trainees gain an insight into the patient's agenda. It is useful if the trainee seems to have a very doctor-centred approach. It is also very useful to aid a trainee in preparing for breaking bad news to a patient. This is an example of how using models in the appropriate context can be quite powerful.

➤ What has happened?
➤ Why has it happened ? Why to me? Why now?
➤ What would happen if I did nothing?
➤ What should I do about it?
➤ What can you (the doctor) do about it?
➤ How can I stop it happening again?

Heron's 1986 six-category intervention analysis

This is a model describing the range of interventions available to the doctor. It is useful when a trainee is having problems in the management of patients – particularly the 'difficult' patient.

➤ Prescriptive – advising/telling.
➤ Informative – instructing/interpreting.
➤ Confronting – challenging/feeding back.
➤ Cathartic – releasing emotions.
➤ Catalytic – encouraging exploration.
➤ Supportive – comforting/affirming.

Berne's 1997 transactional analysis

This is a model of human behaviour (child, adult, parent) and allows an interpretation of some situations which many trainees do find difficult. This first part of his book 'games people play' is an excellent introduction to this.

Murtagh's 1998 model

This, again, is a mechanistic model that has a pragmatic feel to it. It might prove useful to the anxious trainee in that it offers more concrete advice on the uncertainties of diagnosis. Many would feel this was not the ideal solution for dealing with this problem.

➤ What is the probability diagnosis?
➤ What serious diagnosis should not be missed?
➤ What conditions are often missed? (provides a list of conditions)
➤ Is this a 'masquerade'? (provides a list of conditions)
➤ Is the patient trying to tell me something I've missed?

The Cambridge–Calgary model

This adopts an evidence-based approach to consultation skills teaching that will be described later in this section. It has a practical flavour that appeals to many trainers.

➤ Initiating the consultation.

➤ Gathering information.
➤ Building the relationship/facilitating the patient's involvement.
➤ Explanation and planning.
➤ Closing the consultation.

Neighbour's 1987 model

This is widely used by trainers although it is not clear how practical the exercises suggested in the book are in reality. Its attraction seems to lie in the five key words of the model. Summarising, handing over, safety netting and housekeeping seem to have been particularly useful concepts. This will be looked at again later in this chapter.

1 Connecting.
2 Summarising.
3 Handing over.
4 Safety netting.
5 Housekeeping.

Neighbour R. *The Inner Consultation.* Lancaster: Kluwer Academic; 1987 also introduces the idea of 'acceptance sets' and 'calibration sets' and some trainers found this useful. Patients often have particular patterns of body language in response to particular situations. If the doctor can identify the set for agreement (the acceptance set) or other situations (sadness, confusion, frustration, etc.), he can become calibrated to the patient and increase the chance of better communication. Certainly trainers can use the video to illustrate this phenomenon and raise trainee awareness.

Neurolinguistic programming

This has developed a significant following in the US and is quite a complicated system based on models of how the brain handles information. If the communicator can identify the predominant system in the person they are communicating with, then it suggests ways of improving communication with them. Some trainers have found a number of the concepts useful.

➤ Dominant theory states that people view the world from a kinaesthetic (feeling), visual (seeing) or auditory (hearing) point of view. They use and respond to words in their relevant system more readily. They also express their preference in other behaviours, i.e. the visual person will *see* something is wrong and might respond better to a pictorial explanation than a verbal one. If the doctor can use their system they will feel better understood and treated. A particular exercise the trainer can use here is to ask trainees to repeat the advice they gave to the patient but particularly using the patient's own words and trying to use their particular system in some form.

➤ Eye movement indicators are another concept that can be useful. People's eye movements seem to provide insight into thought processes. This is described in detail in Neighbour R. *The Inner Consultation.* Lancaster: Kluwer Academic; 1987. Few people have been able to describe using this on a large scale but it is practical to learn the one or two common movements (i.e. those indicating a feeling or visual memory).

McWhinney's 1972 disease-illness

This model (*see* Figure 7.1) draws a parallel between the traditional medical model of illness and a patient centred perspective. This sort of process may help the trainee with a lot of hospital-based experience as it drafts a patient-centred perspective onto the skeleton of a well-established mode of thinking.

McWhinney, a co-author of the model (with Levenstein 1986), described a dual concept to help understand why a patient presents at a particular time. Patients reach either their 'Limit of symptom tolerance' or their 'Limit of anxiety'. If the doctor can understand which trigger is at work, the consultation is more likely to be successful.

This insight can help focus trainees on the patient agenda.

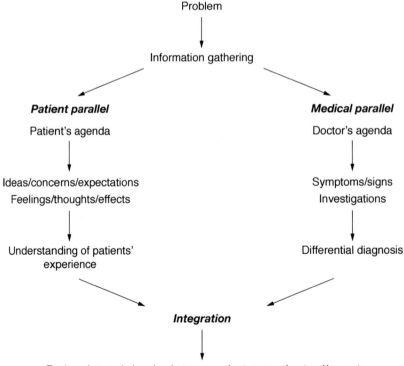

Figure 7.1: McWhinney's disease-illness model.

CONSTRUCTIVE FEEDBACK METHODS

The following are methods for giving constructive feedback in a structured, non-threatening way. Should your practice contain more than one trainee, some trainers find it helpful to facilitate trainees feeding back to each other. This gives the trainer a feel for their feedback and consultation skills while sometimes feeling less threatening than the trainer taking the lead.

Pendleton's rules

These remain a very useful and commonly employed tool. Some would argue that they are a little contrived and that trainees ignore the positive comments ('everything before the but is crap', as someone more crudely put it). However, they are designed to be protective of the learner in a vulnerable situation and it is still the case that many trainees feel threatened by the video. When asking someone to evaluate their own performance, they will usually focus on the negative; this framework ensures they also identify the positives. In summary, the trainer runs through the following scheme after the video consultation.

➤ What do you think you did well?
➤ What do I think you did well?
➤ What do you think you could have done differently? (and how)
➤ What do I think you could have done differently? (and how)
➤ How do you feel about this?
➤ Finish on a positive reinforcement of good consultation behaviour.

The SETGO method

See Kurtz S, Silverman J and Draper J. *Teaching and Learning Communication Skills in Medicine.* Oxford: Radcliffe Medical Press; 1998. We all tend to be our worst critics and this method enables the trainee to identify their own learning goals in a non-threatening way. Its major advantage lies in going straight to the points raised by the learner. Briefly, the trainee and trainer look at the video and make *observational* notes where they think appropriate but generally on a minute-to-minute basis. After the consultation the trainer facilitates the following process.

➤ What did you, the trainee, See?
➤ What Else did I, the trainer, see?
➤ What do you, the trainee, Think about this?
➤ What Goals can we now set?
➤ What Offers have we got to achieve these goals?

i.e. 'SETGO'.

The method then goes on to suggest these offers are role played to give the trainee a chance to develop their skills.

This book contains some very useful lists of generic skills necessary to achieve communication goals. They reduce the communication process down to specific behaviours that are practical to teach, i.e. for building rapport:

➤ demonstrates good eye contact, posture and movement, facial expression and use of voice techniques (language content, modulation)
➤ if the notes or computer are used then it does not interfere with dialogue
➤ acknowledges the patients thoughts and feelings non-judgementally
➤ expresses concern, understanding and willingness to help and acknowledge the patient's coping efforts
➤ deals with sensitive, embarrassing and painful issues sensitively.

The book contains similar lists for all areas of the consultation.

EXAMINATION-BASED METHODS

One of the major drivers of learning is assessment. It would be foolish for trainers to ignore this motivation – and of course they don't.

The MRCGP examination (discussed in more detail in Chapter 3) includes the CSA which in part looks at consultation skills and of course the Consultation Observational Tool (COT).

The marking sheet for the COT can be found at: www.rcgp.org.uk/docs/ MRCGP_COT_Guide_to_Performance_Criteria.doc. In a similar way to some consultation models, this can be reviewed with the trainee to help define a structure for their consultations.

The Clinical Skills Assessment (CSA) will include stations that will in part demand effective use of the consultation – especially as they are strictly timed to 10 minutes. Many trainers will arrange mock CSA cases within the practice. You may also find that these are arranged through the local vocational training scheme. If so, they will often be looking for volunteers to facilitate.

The old-style MRCGP examination included a video component where consultations by the trainee were graded based on a certain criteria. Although this is no longer relevant in terms of examination, the marking guide can again form a way in to help structure the consultation. A copy of the criteria can be found in the learning resource guide.

The RCGP also produces a number of DVDs to help trainees preparing for their exam and for trainers to understand the assessment. These include the following.

➤ *A Guide to the Clinical Skills Assessment* (DVD and workbook). Developed to give candidates an idea of what to expect in the CSA of the new MRCGP examination. Consists of 12 cases chosen to reflect a spectrum of encounters between GP and patient and a workbook with examiners' comments.
➤ *A Guide to the COT of Workplace Based Assessment* (DVD and workbook). The aim of this guide is to help candidates prepare for the COT

assessment, understand the COT's 'performance criteria', and enable trainees to provide the evidence that trainers require when making their judgements. This DVD and handbook are designed to offer practical guidance to trainees and their trainers who must create and adjudge COTs. It advises on how the consultation is assessed, details the performance criteria and analyses each consultation on the DVD with practical advice for each, based on the performance criteria

VIDEO-BASED METHODS

Body language

Many trainers play the video fast forward with the sound off. This highlights problems with body language to trainees. It tends to look amusing, which reduces the threatening element of feedback.

Sex-lives and Videotapes

Matthews P, Skelton J, Wiskin C, Field S. *Sex-Lives and Videotape. Sexual history taking in primary care.* Oxford: Radcliffe Medical Press, 1999 is a video produced by the West Midlands Deanery. It provides an introduction to sexual health and sexual health history taking. Its target audience is a multi-professional one; thus it is a very good tool for GP trainees to use during their training year. It may be difficult to find these days.

Home-made movies

Many trainers have kept videos often of their own consultations, to illustrate certain issues. It seems to de-threaten trainees to show a video 'warts and all' and certainly provides the opportunity for the trainer to show their response to constructive criticism. Come on, put your money where your mouth is . . .

John Cleese and Rob Buckman's videos for patients

These are part of a set of training videos that are very amusing and provoke discussion. More information can be found at: www.videosforpatients.co.uk/ Products.html.

Other videos

Elsewhere in this book we have a list of resources including multimedia clips that can be used to illustrate communication techniques (*see* Chapter 8).

JOINT SURGERIES/VISITS

This was the second most common method used to assess and teach consulting skills. In Australia it is the primary teaching method and is favoured for its immediacy. It has problems relating to time, the distortion of consultation dynamics and reduction of service time within the practice. Some trainers overcome the problem of distortion by sitting in the next room and having the consultation filmed 'live'. Use of Pendleton's rules and role play are useful in a debrief after the consultation. Where it does have advantages is in the role modelling demonstration of skills by the trainer and in the opportunity for the trainer to intervene in real time with a real patient. Trainees often comment positively on this and it may be an under-used tool in the UK system.

Some trainers suggested using Saturday mornings or half days for this to relieve the time pressure.

ROLE PLAY

This is used commonly by trainers. It can be difficult to introduce with some trainees but many enjoy the fun element of it. It can be a safe way to explore some communication problem areas, i.e. the angry patient, the confrontation, the breaking of bad news. Some trainers use scenarios from Drucquer M, Hutchinson S. *The Consultation Toolkit: a practical method for teaching and learning consultation skills*. Surrey: Reed Healthcare Publishing; 2000. A useful resource in these situations can be a sheet of desirable behaviours that can be referred to and then practised. These instructions can usefully be developed as the initial part of the tutorial between the trainer and the trainee and then role played with the final backup of the resource sheets. This is the basis of Barrows H, Tamblyn R. *Problem-Based Learning: An Approach to Medical Education*. New York: Springer Publishing Company; 1980.

➤ Problem: the trainee needs to tell someone bad news.
➤ Questions: (generated by the trainee in the tutorial or in preparation).
➤ Solutions: (generated by trainee with facilitation).
➤ Role play of solutions.
➤ Assessment of what works well.
➤ Refer to resource sheet to ensure no major areas missed.
➤ Arrange to look at areas missed (if any) and review use of new skills.

Kurtz S, Silverman J and Draper J. *Skills for Communicating with Patients*. Oxford: Radcliffe Medical Press; 1998 has excellent sections covering core skills in all areas of communication including confrontation and breaking bad news. These make good resource sheets for this sort of exercise.

A particular exercise mentioned for role play was the 'option-raising exercise'. This is useful for the trainee who, often having taken a thorough history considering the patient's agenda well, switches back to a medical doctor-centred model and proceeds to tell the patient what to do. It appears many trainees feel patients expect them to 'behave like a doctor' when it comes to management and they give prescriptive advice. In this exercise the trainer role plays a patient (preferably one from the trainees experience) and the trainee is asked to deliberately discuss ALL the options for management with the trainer. The trainer can use the opportunity to demonstrate the effect patient health beliefs can have on management and help develop negotiation and sharing skills.

Neighbour R. *The Inner Consultation*. Lancaster: Kluwer Academic; 1987 contains a number of other exercises that can be used in this manner or explored in the consultation itself.

Another exercise mentioned could be described as the RCGP model exercise – as mentioned previously, the RCGP model simply states that problems have a physical, social and psychological element. Despite the obvious nature of this to GPs many candidates for the MRCGP do not seem to enquire into this area. If this appears to be a problem the trainer can role play presentations from the trainee's notes, video or e-portfolio using the 'filter' that the trainee must ask some questions that look at these areas. The trainer can try and introduce points that have a bearing on the presentation. This can then be followed by a discussion on how this would influence the consultation for both the doctor and the patient (*see* BATHE exercise in Chapter 9).

TUTORIAL-BASED EXERCISES

A number of these were mentioned by trainers. Generally, they are methods that tackle particular problems that have emerged with trainees, and are done in pairs with the trainer.

Listening skills exercise

This is useful where there is evidence that the trainee is perhaps interrupting or not listening to the patient. The trainee is asked to describe a particular event (i.e. most useful learning experience, best holiday, etc.) and the trainer demonstrates 'active listening'. There is then a discussion where the learner identifies the components of active listening and the roles are reversed. A variant is for the trainer deliberately to demonstrate the opposite skills (destructive listening?). The trainer then summarises by reinforcing the relevant skills. The whole process can be video-taped to allow better review.

Empathic language exercise

This is useful where the trainee appears to be using personal language constructs inappropriately with patients (often very medicalised complex language). This probably impedes development of rapport. The trainee is asked to describe an event that has some emotional content for them for two or three minutes. The trainer summarises this twice: first, using different words and with interpretation and, secondly, using the trainee's language content and reflection. After a discussion about how this felt for the trainee, the trainer describes a similar event and the trainee summarises this using the trainer's language and reflection. The trainer then reinforces the new skills demonstrated.

Many more of these type of exercises are described in Burnard P. *Teaching Interpersonal Skills*. London: Chapman and Hall; 1991.

Telephone consultations

Consultations that eliminate the 'face-to-face' element are becoming increasingly more commonplace whether in everyday surgery or sessions with the out-of-hours co-operative. Some trainers will therefore look specifically at the skills required in this area. There are useful tips and scenarios on the Bradford VTS website at: www.bradfordvts.co.uk. Methods include role playing with both patient and doctor sitting facing away from each other or 'piggy backing' real phone calls, so that the trainer can listen in on what the trainee is saying, or even phoning each other on the practice internal call system. One of the great advantages of this is that is stops trainees making assumptions based simply on a patient's appearance, so they really have to use their consulting skills to develop a picture in their mind of the patient's current state.

SUMMARY

Consultation skills can be one of the most fascinating areas to teach during the training year. Trainers have differing opinions in consultation models but they can be extremely useful to identify where a trainee may be having difficulties. Direct observation through video and joint surgeries can be invaluable but be prepared to put yourself on the line in order to make it less threatening. The ongoing task is to balance the 'here' (i.e. what they need to learn to pass exams) with the future (i.e. what skills will see them through the next 30 years)!

There is an interesting dichotomy between the type of teaching method that uses an intuitive process and that using a logical process. Some would say this relates to the hemispheric cerebral dominance inherent in the assessor, i.e. you are left dominant so logical, rational and controlled (the scientist) or right dominant and creative, intuitive and spontaneous (the artist). Both approaches have value that need to be acknowledged and it is probably a mistake to use either exclusively. This chapter has offered practical approaches for consultation skills teaching for each of your cerebral hemispheres and some that may even involve both!

CHAPTER 8

Resources: what resources do trainers use?

Where shall I find all the time to do this non-reading? (Krauss)

WHAT INFORMATION TECHNOLOGY, BOOKS AND REFERENCE SOURCES ARE TRAINERS USING?

Introduction

Many trainers are hoarders – they keep collections of references, pictures, slides, tapes, websites and props of all sorts. These are very individual collections and are sometimes used and sometimes not. Some trainers dislike this approach. This section offers suggestions that may be useful. It will often be ideal for the trainee to search for their own references but life is life, people are people and these resources may be more pragmatic at times.

Most of the items in this list of references have proved useful over a number of years. Some will date but usually they relate to the principles or the process in that area, or are considered important or 'seminal' work.

We believe all the references and resources are described in sufficient detail for trainers to find or order them. Some items may be out of publication – established trainers can be a useful source of these.

The advent of the internet means we can all find 'data' whenever we want, but finding 'information' may be a bit more challenging – most of us understand this difference which is often demonstrated by patients carrying internet printouts! The first part of this section lists the books trainers find useful in specific circumstances and we have tried to tie these into the new curriculum where possible. The second part identifies websites trainers find useful. The third lists references, films and other ideas trainers have found useful: many of the older articles still have seminal lessons to teach.

The doubling time of total available knowledge is an interesting concept. It probably took 50 years for the total of all world knowledge to double at the turn of the century. By the 1950s it was about five years, in 1980 about three months and now it is estimated in days. How long before it is in hours, minutes or even seconds? With this rate of progression it is difficult to see how the printed word can keep up! Doctors need to be able to access salient information and to work with a 'playable hand' of this data. Future generations will have to learn to cope with this problem, perhaps without books – but we are not there yet. This section describes the books trainers recommend. There should be enough detail to order or find the book.

General advice

Patterns of reading habits vary enormously. Some doctors seem to read very little and remain well informed using other methods. Some doctors read extensively and seem relatively uninformed. Others seem to acquire a vast data of knowledge but possess little wisdom. Some stand out as both knowledgeable and wise.

Many trainees have developed poor reading habits. They seem to fall into a number of patterns (*see* Table 8.1).

Table 8.1

'All or nothing reading'	The trainee thinks they should read everything! Anyone who seriously tries this will end up reading nothing. Some seem to start at the nothing level.
'Biblical reading'	The trainee is determined to find a book that will answer all their worries. This can work at the undergraduate medicine level but not in primary care.
'Binge reading'	The trainee reads in patches but has no regular habit and usually resents the process, i.e. it is done for tutorial preparation, exams or presentations only.
'Comfort reading'	The trainee tends to read about areas they already know and avoids other areas, providing a false sense of reassurance and security.

The trainer can facilitate the evolution of a good reading habit in many ways. It is generally accepted that the retention of knowledge from reading is maximised by spending at least an equal (if not greater) time deliberately recalling/rehearsing new learning as the time spent actually reading. The role modelling approach is helpful by demonstrating a positive attitude to reading. Pragmatic advice can be given – *see* www.radcliffepublishing.com/gptrainershandbook for an example of an advice sheet for trainees. The concepts of reflective learning can be used to focus the trainee to read relevant areas related to their experience. Finally the trainer can suggest (or even directly supply) the book to be read.

BOOKS

The practice library

What books should a training practice have in the their library? Many trainers have asked themselves this question – usually just before a training practice accreditation visit! It is really the wrong question – the modern approach is about 'knowledge management' – can trainees access the knowledge they need, when they need it in a form they need?

However, arguably, some books still have some roles:

➤ to act as a reference source for the PHCT that is up to date, accessible and user-friendly
➤ to act as a stimulus to the development of the practice and individuals
➤ to satisfy any external assessors.

One method of assessing the library can be found at: www.radcliffepublishing. com/gptrainershandbook This is a tool used by visiting teams on training accreditation visits and can be used by trainers to assess their own libraries – bearing in mind the role of IT.

Trainers should consider a written library policy to cover the following areas:

➤ named member of PHCT in charge
➤ named clerical support staff
➤ a catalogue system that lists books by title/author/subject/date of publication (plus ISBN number/publisher if desired)
➤ a defined and easily recognised filing system
➤ a policy for lending books and recording their whereabouts/spotting unreturned books
➤ a policy for periodic review of contents, i.e. for weeding out and adding to the library
➤ a policy on acquiring and cataloguing new books
➤ a budgetary policy for the library
➤ an advertising process to raise awareness of new material to the readership
➤ a process to review and audit the library policy
➤ a policy for dealing with journals (i.e. which ones/how long to be kept, etc.)
➤ a system for storing and displaying material that is difficult to classify (i.e. NHS documents, folders, videos, IT resources, tapes, etc.).

The list of books in Table 8.2 was considered recommended reading by trainers. The list can be used to identify recommended books in specific areas and we have suggested a potential link to the curriculum statements. We haven't read them all so you might like to fill in some gaps!

Table 8.2 Books

We are 'signposting' these books and believe we have provided enough (albeit scanty) detail that will allow trainers to find them and encourage their 'search skills'.

Title	Author(s) and publisher	Comments	Curriculum link
Practical General Practice	Khot and Polmear	A very concise, well set out 'starter'	Clinical management
Symptom sorter	Hopcroft and Forte	A useful symptom-based book for the surgery	Clinical management
The Oxford Handbook of Emergencies in General Practice	Lawrence et al		Clinical management
The Oxford Textbook of General Practice	Simon and Everitt		Clinical management
An Atlas of Dermatology	Lots – take your choice but also see the website list		Clinical management
The Man who Mistook his Wife for a Hat	Sacks	Fascinating neurological presentations	Clinical management
'At a Glance' DVLA guidance on fitness to drive	DVLA		Clinical management
Contraception: Your Questions Answered Contraception Today: a pocketbook for primary care practitioners	Guillebaud	Still regarded as the most useful texts in this area	Clinical management
Rheumatology Guidelines	Ferarri, Cash and Martin		Clinical management
The ABC series	BMJ Books		Clinical management
The Oxford Textbook of Medicine	Warell, Cox and Firth		Clinical management
The One Minute Manager The One Minute Manager Meets the Monkey	Blanchard	Coffee-time reading but still very illuminating on management and delegation	Working with colleagues

Title	Author(s) and publisher	Comments	Curriculum link
Developing Teamwork	Goldsmith and Kindred	A short book on teams – uses Myers Briggs model	Working with colleagues
Once upon a Team	Kindred and Kindred	A book of team exercises	Working with colleagues
The Inner Consultation	Neighbour	Fairly lengthy but has a number of useful exercises and the overall model is very practical	Communication and consulting skills
Clean Language: revealing metaphors and opening minds	Sullivan and Rees	For the more astute trainee (and trainer!)	Communication and consulting skills
The Doctor's Communication Handbook	Tate	Very concise over-view – highly recommended	Communication and consulting skills
The Doctor, His Patient and the Illness	Balint	A seminal, rather difficult read – find a shorter summary unless you really have time!	Communication and consulting skills
Games People Play	Berne	A very useful description of patient behaviours that can enlighten trainees	Communication and consulting skills
Skills for Communicating with Patients	Silverman, Kurtz and Draper	A detailed system with many useful pointers	Communication and consulting skills
How to Break Bad News	Buckman	Considered an excellent over-view	Communication and consulting skills
Principles of NLP	O'Connor	An introductory text really	Communication and consulting skills
The New Consultation: developing doctor-patient communication	Pendleton et al	A reworking of the original classic	Communication and consulting skills
Learning to Consult	Charlton	A very useful, practical approach	Communication and consulting skills
Metaphors We Live By	Lakoff	Perhaps for the more astute trainees	Communication and consulting skills
An Introduction to NLP	O'Connor	Now a more detailed guide to using NLP	Communication and consulting skills

Title	Author(s) and publisher	Comments	Curriculum link
I'm OK You're OK	Harris	A useful model to look at human interactions	Communication and consulting skills
Families and How to Survive Them	Cleese and Skynner	A humorous look at family behaviours	Communication and consulting skills
Love's Executioner	Yalom	A good read about more in-depth therapeutic relationships	Communication and consulting skills
How to Read a Paper	Greenhlagh	A well-established leader in this area	Data gathering and interpretation
Bad Science	Goldacre	A very readable paperback – evidence-based medicine in the real world	Making a diagnosis/making decisions
Irrationality	Sutherland	This book is quite hard work at times but full of interesting studies exposing the elements of decision-making	Making a diagnosis/making decisions
Reckoning with Risk	Gigerenzer	A bit mathematical but still a good read on risk	Making a diagnosis/making decisions
The Art of General Practice	Morell	Widens perspectives on the role	Managing medical complexity
The Mystery of General Practice	Heath	An inspiring book from an inspiring author	Managing medical complexity
The Paradox of Progress	Willis	Broadens understanding of how the medical world operates	Managing medical complexity
Complexity for Clinicians	Holt and Marinker	Brings the issues of complexity theory into context	Managing medical complexity
A Fortunate Man: the story of a country doctor	Berger	A real challenge to our values as doctors	Community orientation
Leaves from the Life of a Country Doctor	Buchan and Gunn	An interesting look at working in general practice	Community orientation
A Country Doctor's Notebook	Bulgakov and Glenny	More insights – life as a GP	Community orientation
The Art of War	Sun Tzu and Manford	2000 years old and full of insights into human behaviour	Practicing holistically

Title	Author(s) and publisher	Comments	Curriculum link
Darkness Visible	Styron	A personal and very brief description of depression	Practicing holistically
The Diving Bell and the Butterfly	Bauby	An inspiring story of locked-in syndrome	Practicing holistically
I Never Promised you a Rose Garden	Greenberg	Insights regarding schizophrenia	Practicing holistically
The Book of Lost Things	Connolly	Dementia	Practicing holistically
The Savage God	Alvrez	Suicide	Practicing holistically
Iris: a memoir of Iris Murdoch	Bayley	Dementia	Practicing holistically
On Death and Dying	Kubler-Ross E		Practicing holistically
Because Cowards Get Cancer Too	Diamond	A personal account	Practicing holistically
The Island	Hislop		Practicing holistically
Lucky	Seebold	About rape	Practicing holistically
Through Grief: the bereavement journey	Collick	Grief	Practicing holistically
My Left Foot	Brown C		Practicing holistically
A Grief Observed	Lewis CS	Grief	Practicing holistically
Trainspotting	Welsh	Drug use and abuse	Practicing holistically
The Curious Incident of the Dog in the Night-time	Haddon	Autism insights	Practicing holistically
The BMA Handbook of Medical Ethics	BMJ Books	A standard text	Maintaining an ethical approach
The Peaceable Kingdom: a primer in Christian ethics	Hauerwas	Interesting discussion areas	Maintaining an ethical approach
Playing God	Bullough	A challenge to our role as GPs	Maintaining an ethical approach
BNF			Maintaining performance, learning and teaching
The Seven Habits of Highly Effective People	Covey	A useful model of effective behaviours	Maintaining performance, learning and teaching
The Tao of Pooh	Hoff and Shepherd	An interesting insight into 'typing' people – what would Milne have thought!	Maintaining performance, learning and teaching

Title	Author(s) and publisher	Comments	Curriculum link
Feel the Fear and Do it Anyway	Jeffers		Maintaining performance, learning and teaching
The Tipping Point	Gladwell		Maintaining performance, learning and teaching
The GP Trainers Handbook	Middleton and Field	A tool box for trainers	Maintaining performance, learning and teaching
The Inner Apprentice	Neighbour	An excellent view of training by a major contributor to the profession	Maintaining performance, learning and teaching
Teaching for Quality Education at University	Biggs	Some useful theory and practice	Maintaining performance, learning and teaching
The Concise GP Curriculum	RCGP publication		Maintaining performance, learning and teaching
Medical Education	Fish and Coles	An overview	Maintaining performance, learning and teaching
Teaching and Learning Consultation Skills in Medicine	Silverman, Kurtz and Draper	Full of practical advice	Maintaining performance, learning and teaching
Once Upon a Group	Kindred	A short manual of group behaviours – good for group teachers	Maintaining performance, learning and teaching
Essential MRCGP CSA Preparation and Practice Cases	Knight	MRCGP	Maintaining performance, learning and teaching
Notes for the MRCGP	Palmer and Boekx	MRCGP	Maintaining performance, learning and teaching
The Complete MRCGP Study Guide	Gear	MRCGP	Maintaining performance, learning and teaching
EMQs for the MRCGP Applied Knowledge Test	Dawson and Trigell	MRCGP	Maintaining performance, learning and teaching
StrengthsFinder 2.0 Develop Self-awareness Now, Discover Your Learning Strengths	Rath (Gallup)		Maintaining performance, learning and teaching

WEBSITES

> To err is human, to Google divine (apologies to Alexander Pope)

Trainers now have to use IT resources in teaching – and trainees usually have a higher level of competence in IT use than their trainers! The DOH expects all healthcare professionals to have the following competencies:

1 to use IT facilities in the consultation (prescribing, note keeping, reviews, etc.)
2 to be able to access medical literature online (using pubmed, medline – *see* at: http://primarycarelearninghub.hfac.keele.ac.uk/cpd/ for an advice sheet on how to acquire an Athens number)
3 to be able to send and receive e-mail communications
4 to be able to use search engines to find data on the internet
5 to use IT facilities in decision support in the consultation.

The final area above involves clinical support systems available to advise on clinical care guidelines, prescribing and referral criteria and even diagnostic decision support. Many current systems already have under-used decision support systems (e.g. Emis and mentor project) which have educational potential.

Some experts believe all this will be available on mobile phone-sized, voice-activated devices within 10 years. Professor Kidd has coined the five 'golden rules' of IT.

Rule 1 IT is *not* always the answer.
Rule 2 IT solutions are expensive.
Rule 3 Remember to look outside your own hard disc for a source of help.
Rule 4 The internet is full of disorganised data *not* information.
Rule 5 Sometimes IT is essential.

We should be aiming to learn *about* IT, learn *through* IT and learn *with* IT.

Woods and trees come to mind as far as the internet is concerned and the trick is to find a 'good site'. Many of these are referred to throughout the book. Table 8.3 pulls these together and adds a few more.

Table 8.3 Websites

Site URL	Notes
www.gpnotebook.com	A very useful source of information – has educational material as well.
http://resources.scalingtheheights.com	This site is a rich source of well-established material to support trainers and the more 'cutting' edge stuff too – a well established and respected 'teaching the teachers' organisation.

Site URL	Notes
www.unco.edu/cetl/sir/stating_outcome/documents/Krathwohl.pdf	Revised version of Bloom's cognitive domain.
www.rcgp-curriculum.org.uk/PDF/curr_1_Curriculum_Statement_Being_a_GP.pdf	
www.rcgp-curriculum.org.uk/rcgp_-_gp_curriculum_documents/gp_curriculum_statements.aspx	The RCGP curriculum statement sites.
www.rcgp-curriculum.org.uk	
www.rcgp-curriculum.org.uk/extras/curriculum	
www.gp-training.net/training/assessment/formative/nmrs/index.htm	New Manchester Rating Scales.
www.gp-training.net/training/tools/nnr.htm	New Northumberland Rating Scales.
http://cms.rcgp.org.uk/gpcurriculum/docs/Condensed%20Curriculum%20Guide%20-%20self-assessment%20scale.xls	RCGP confidence rating scale.
www.rcgp-curriculum.org.uk/PDF/curr_The_Learning_and_Teaching_Guide_dec08.pdf	RCGP Learning and Teaching Guide.
www.e-gp.org	RCGP interactive e-learning resource.
www.rcgp-innovait.oxfordjournals.org	The AiT journal site.
www.gmc-uk.org/static/documents/content/GMC_GMP_0911.pdf	The GMC document link.
www.woncaeurope.org/Web%20documents/European%20Definition%20of%20family%20medicine/Definition%20EURACTshort%20version.pdf	The WONCA link.
www.bradfordvts.co.uk	This site is incredible! It has concise advice sheets on everything and every trainer should visit it.
www.westmidlandsdeanery.nhs.uk/LinkClick.aspx?fileticket=2Zf9yHHuSvg%3d&tabid=170&mid=898	A guide for educational supervisors.
www.gp-training.net	This site has a wide range of educational material.
www.rcgp.org.uk/docs/MRCGP_How%20to%20plan%20and%20conduct%20the%20CBD%20interview.doc	Guidance for CbD.
www.rcgp.org.uk/docs/MRCGP_CBD%20Structured%20Question%20Guidance.doc	
www.rcgp.org.uk/docs/MRCGP_COT_Guide_to_Performance_Criteria.doc.	Guidance for COT.
www.rcgp.org.uk/docs/MRCGP_msf%20form%20from%20e-portfolio.doc	The MSF document.

Site URL	Notes
www.rcgp.org.uk/Docs/MRCGP_all%20six%20 assessment%20forms.doc	The PSQ document.
http://distributedresearch.net/wiki/index.php/ Gibbs_reflective_Cycle	The Gibbs reflective cycle site.
www.peterhoney.com/content/ LearningStylesQuestionnaire.html	The Learning style site.
www.learning-styles-online.com/	An overview of learning styles.
www.eguidelines.co.uk	
http://dorakmt.tripod.com/mtd/glosstat.html	Statistical definitions.
www.passmedicine.com	MRCGP sites.
www.oneexamination.com	
www.pastest.co.uk	
www.pennine-gp-training.co.uk	This site has a number of useful advice
www.pennine-gp-training.co.uk/Ed-Sup-RCGP-Form.doc	sheets for supervisors.
http://resources.scalingtheheights.com/ wolverhampton_grid.htm	Wolverhampton grid.
www.npep.org.uk/	The nPEP site.
www.rcgp.org.uk/professional_development/ essential_knowledge_updates.aspx	The RCGP EKU site – with excellent educational links to the areas covered.
http://primarycarelearninghub.hfac.keele.ac.uk/ cpd/	This site is aimed at the West Midlands but also contains an index of websites.
www.belbin.com	The Belbin team style site.
www.businessballs.com/personalitystylesmodels. htm	A great site with all sorts of educational resources – this one on personality styles.
http://careers.d.umn.edu/inventories/personality_ test_intro.html	Personality style inventory.
www.personalitypathways.com/type_inventory. html	Myers-Briggs site.
www.the-mdu.com/	
womenshealthinbrightonandsussex.org.uk	
www.healthtalkonline.org/	An excellent site with podcasts of patient experiences.
www.skillscascade.com/index.html	A Cambridge site devoted to communication skills.
www.nice.org.uk/	Guideline sites.
www.sign.ac.uk/	
www.medicine.ox.ac.uk/bandolier/	
www2.cochrane.org/reviews/	

Site URL	Notes
www.patient.co.uk/ www.equip.nhs.uk/	Sites to inform patients – patient UK has excellent leaflets.
http://learning.bmj.com/learning/main.html http://podcasts.bmj.com/	The BMJ sites – good quality and comprehensive.
www.healthcarerepublic.com/	A comprehensive site with information and education material.
www.univadis.co.uk/medical_and_more/UK_Login_search	A developing site with a lot of educational material – and an excellent anatomy section.
www.gpehub.org/	Based at Warwick University and contains resources targeted at trainees and trainers.
http://dermnetnz.org/	A New Zealand site with excellent dermatology resources.
www.npci.org.uk/	A brilliant virtual 'building' – excellent resources to support any prescribing teaching and learning.
www.mtrac.co.uk/	Advice and independent assessment for the use of medicines.
www.cks.nhs.uk/home	Easy to search clinical knowledge summaries covering many areas.
www.doctors.net.uk/	A comprehensive site with educational material.
www.cdc.gov/ www.hpa.org.uk/	Communicable diseases site Health Protection Agency.
www.mapofmedicine/com	The Map of Medicine is a valuable tool for healthcare professionals. Because it is underpinned by NICE guidance, where this is available, it supports our commitment to encourage implementation of our guidance and encourage evidence-based practice in healthcare. It is a free site with a lot of educational content.
www.medscape.com	This is the American combination of gpnotebook and the NPCI type site with online educational tutorials as well as a full database of American-based resources – very good.

REFERENCES FOR TRAINEES

Table 8.4

Asthma		
	BTS guidelines	
	Diagnosis	*BMJ.* editorial 5 July 1997
Cardiology		
	Use of ECG in diagnosis of heart failure	*BMJ.* January 1996
Cholesterol		
	Scandinavian Simvastatin Survival Study	*Lancet.* November 1994
	CARE	*NEJM.* 1996
	West of Scotland coronary prevention study	*BMJ.* 1997; **315**: 7122
	Heartsink patients	*BMJ.* 1988; **297**: 20–7
	The difficult doctor/patient relationship: somatisation, personality and psychopathology	*J Clin Epidemiol.* 1994; **47**(6: 647–57
	Empathy: an essential skill for understanding the physician/patient relationship in clinical practice	*Fam Med.* 1993; **25**(4): 245–8
	Doctor/patient relationship: Toronto consensus	*J Gen Intern Med.* 1988; **3**: 177–90
Evidence-based medicine		
	Socratic dissent	*BMJ.* 1995; **310**: 1126–7
	EBM – an approach to clinical problem solving	*BMJ.* 1995; **310**: 1122–6
Ethics		
	Four principles plus scope	*BMJ.* 16 July 1994
	Drug representative visits	*BMJ.* May 1996
Investigations/ diagnosis		
	Use of the normal investigation to reassure	*BMJ.* 18 August 1996
	There's a lot of it about: clinical strategies in family practice	*BJGP.* 1986; **36**: 468–71
	Problem solving and decision-making in family practice	*Can Fam Phys.*1979; **25**: 1473
Paediatrics		
	Listen to parents: they know best	*BMJ.* 1996; **313**: 954–5
	What worries parents when their pre-school children are acutely ill and why?	*BMJ.* 1996; **313**: 983–6

Professional development		
	Life, your career and the pursuit of happiness	*BMJ classified*. 25 Oct 1997; 2
Psychiatry/ Neurology		
	How to perform a rapid neurological examination	*Update*. 1 Oct 1997
	Unrecognised psychiatric illness in primary care	*BJGP*. June 1996
Referrals		
	The gatekeeper and the wizard	*BMJ*. 1989; **298**: 172–4
	The gatekeeper and the wizard revisited	*BMJ*. 1992; **304**: 969–71
Screening		
	Screening can damage your health	*BMJ editorial*. February 1997
Teenagers		
	Sex and risk taking	*BMJ*. 1993; **307**: 25
Palliative care		
	I desperately needed to see my son	*BMJ*. 1991; **302**: 356
	An open letter to my surgeon	*BMJ*. 1992; **305**: 62

* Papers that particularly lend themselves to a tutorial with a critical appraisal element.

REFERENCES FOR TRAINERS

The list in Table 8.5 includes references trainers have found useful in developing their own teaching skills. We are 'signposting' these articles and believe we have provided enough detail that will allow trainers to find them and encourage their 'search skills'.

Table 8.5

Learning by reflection	*Education for General Practice*. 1995; **7**: 237–48
The emotional diary: a framework for reflective learning	*Education for General Practice*. 1997; **8**: 288–91
Personal construct analysis	*Education for General Practice*. 1993; **2**: 121–25
Role modelling: a case study in general practice	*Medical Education*. 1992; **26**: 116–22
The continuum of problem-based learning	*Medical Teacher*. 1998; **20**: 317
Motivation and continuation of professional development	*BJGP*. 1998; **48**: 1429–32.
Independent learning among GP trainees: an initial survey	*Medical Education*. 1992; **26**: 497–502

How we teach key aspects of GP	*Medical Teacher.* 1991; **1**: 93
Avoiding the myths: a pre-requisite for teaching ethics	*Education for General Practice.* 1992; **3**: 117–24
Assessment of trainer performance in RCA	*Education for General Practice.* 1998; **9**: 199–202
Pathologies of 1:1 teaching	*Education for General Practice.* 1996; **7**: 118–22
The S-SDRLS: a short questionnaire about self-directed learning	*Education for General Practice.* 1993; **4**: 121–5
Dudek NL, Marks MB, Regehr G. Failure to fail: the perspectives of clinical supervisors	*Education for Primary Care.* 2006; **17**(1): 81–5
Gillespie, M. Student-teacher connection: a place of possibility	*Journal of Advanced Nursing.* 2005; **52**(2): 211–9

Most of these articles come from three postgraduate medical education journals. Most trainers found *Education for Primary Care* (the 'Green Journal') the most relevant. Details of all three are shown in Table 8.6.

Table 8.6

Education for Primary Care	www.radcliffe-oxford.com/journals/J02_Education_for_ Primary Care/default.htm
Medical Education	www.mededuc.com
Medical Teacher	www.medicalteacher.org/

The Association for Medical Education is another organisation trainers may find useful – *see* at: www.asme.org.uk/

OTHER RESOURCES

➤ *Effective consulting – the five key tasks.* Tate's DVD for trainees and established doctors (not specifically CSA orientated).
➤ *Consulting: communication skills for GPs in training.* A RCGP DVD particularly for trainees doing the MRCGP.
➤ *Say the right thing.* A video from BBC for Business BBC Worldwide Ltd, 1995, on assertive language – one of a number of videos available from http://resources.glos.ac.uk/departments/personnel/staffdev/resources.cfm
➤ **Anatomical models**
  – Commercial models for joint injection of the shoulder, knee and wrist are expensive to buy but can be borrowed from Ciba-Geigy via the local representative.
  – Some practices own or borrow resuscitation dummies (candidates for the MRCGP must submit a CPR competency certificate from an accredited CPR trainer).

➤ **Films**: The following films have some potential for use in training (many of these are taken from the UBC Residents handbook):
  - 'Dad' – a son connecting with a dying father
  - 'Long days journey into night' – alcoholism
  - 'One flew over the cuckoo's nest' – mental illness
  - 'The best little girl in town' – anorexia
  - 'Nothing in common' – divorce and families
  - 'Whose life is it anyway' – paraplegia/assisted suicide
  - 'A duet for one' – a musician with MS
  - 'Sex, lies and videotapes' – sexuality
  - 'Saving Private Ryan' – look for the brief section where he breaks bad news to the wrong 'Private Ryan' – try using the guidelines to assess Tom Hanks' skills
  - 'The Dead Poets Society' – this has a number of scenes that can be useful particularly in the 'teaching to teach' scenario.

For those with a really keen interest, try Stuart M, *et al. Cinemeducation: A Comprehensive Guide to Using Film in Medical Education.* Oxford: Radcliffe Publishing; 2004.

➤ **Poetry**
  - Laing R. *The Knot.* London: Random House; 1970.
  - Colquhuon G. *Playing God: poems about medicine.* London: Hammersmith Press; 2007.
  - Kipling R. 'I keep six honest serving men'.

➤ **Art**
  - 'The Doctor' by Fildes
  - Google 'gout' images and look for a black Imp!
  - An interesting book to consider here is Barritt P. *Humanity in Healthcare: the heart and soul of medicine.* Oxford: Radcliffe Publishing; 2005.
  - The Scaling the Heights website has a section that adds to this list – but trainers can, and often do, use their own imagination here! *See* at: www.resources.scalingtheheights.com/link_arts_supplement.htm
  - Try using topical newspaper cuttings, music, YouTube, Google images. *See* Powley E and Higson R. *The Arts in Medical Education.* Oxford: Radcliffe Publishing; 2005, which enlarges this area.

SUMMARY

> A bad workman blames his tools. (Anon)

If the quotation is true, then perhaps the good workmen is equally appreciative of his tools. Despite this trainers need to keep an eye open for a number of pitfalls: the favourite tool doesn't do every job; in other words, be careful that the teaching is learner-centred and not simply for the trainer's amusement! Don't use a hammer for every job or, as one trainer put it, 'don't go into auto-pilot'. Trainers need to reflect on the appropriateness and usefulness of their teaching methods and beware of trotting out last year's 'lesson'. However, good workmen employ a range of tools for a range of tasks and this chapter describes some of the resources trainers use.

CHAPTER 9

Education gems: trainers' 'tips and tricks'

. . . ideas are born from life. (Weizsacker)

WHAT OTHER IDEAS DID TRAINERS HAVE TO SHARE?

When completing the questionnaire, many trainers added comments and shared thoughts that do not fit easily into the other chapters. It would be a shame to lose them so here they are; some are the 'after-dinner mints' of the manual (short and sweet), others are the cheese and port (food for thought and appreciation) and some perhaps even the party games (frivolous and fun).

We have tried to link them to the competency framework – but it's a pretty loose link!

TRAINERS' EDUCATIONAL GEMS

Clinical management

ABCD

This is a aide-memoir to think about when facing an ill child. It helps to analyse the components of the seriously ill child presentation (*see* Table 9.1).

Table 9.1 ABCD

Alertness	**A**tony	**A**ge-related responsiveness
Breathing (especially recession)		
Circulation	**C**rying (wimper)	**C**oncern (parental)
Diet (i.e. reduced or none)	**D**ehydration	

(Modified from Hewson P and Gollan R. A simple hospital triaging system for infants with acute illness. *J Paed Child Health*.1995; **31**: 29–32.) It can form the basis for a tutorial or analysis of a clinical situation.

Admission

Many trainees have negative feelings about admitting patients, that have their roots in the derogatory comments made by hospital doctors on the receiving end of an admission. Discussing this issue can help, but the following four-point 'reasons for admission' can be a useful means of considering the issues.

Medical	The patient's medical condition alone justifies admission.
Social	The social situation at home, combined with the clinical problem, makes admission advisable.
Organisational	Although this situation could be managed at home, the system cannot meet the needs of this patient (e.g. your home physiotherapy service is unavailable in this area).
Personal	Your personal feelings or circumstances make managing this patient at home difficult (e.g. you're going on holiday tonight).

CAGE

This is a screening tool to help trainees enquire about alcohol consumption. Has anyone Criticised the patient about their consumption? Does it Annoy them when people enquire about their consumption? Do they feel Guilty about their intake? and Do they drink early in the morning (Eye-opener)? Two or more positive answers suggest alcohol dependence.

AUDIT-C

Many find this a more user-friendly tool than FAST: *see* at: www.hepatitis. va.gov/vahep?page=prtop03-audit_c#S1X or just google AUDIT-C

Minor surgery tips

1 You can practice excision of cysts by pushing an olive under loosened pork skin (get a knuckle from the butcher) and trying to excise it without marking the olive (i.e. you wouldn't have broken the cyst).
2 Make a video of your own/your partner's minor operations to use in demonstration of technique.
3 Xanthelasma can be treated with 20% or 40% potassium hydroxide. The lower strength is painted on very carefully (to avoid the eye) with a cotton wool bud. The lesion turns a dramatic white and then involutes. The treatment can be repeated with the higher strength if necessary.
4 Produce a list of procedures to be 'ticked off' as they are done. This tends to ensure that most procedures are kept in mind and covered.

Working with colleagues and in teams

Settling a trainee in

The following touches were suggested by one trainer:

➤ make sure a nameplate is up on their room and give it to them when they leave

➤ ask them to bring in some pictures in the first week
➤ give them a box of equipment and the important paperwork and the time to go and put it in their room where they want it
➤ put a brief description on the notice board, telling patients a bit about them
➤ do a paperchase around the practice with a task/quiz at each location.

Job interviews

A number of resources were suggested:
➤ try visiting www.howto.co.uk/careers/questions-at-interview/
➤ find the series of articles from BMJ careers:
  - What not to do in an interview. *BMJ: Career Focus.* 13 August 2005; 65–6
  - Dressing the part. *BMJ: Career Focus.* 13 August 2005; 67
  - Fair interviewing is harder than it looks. *BMJ: Career Focus.* 13 August 2005; 68–9
  - The research fellow interview. *BMJ: Career Focus.* 13 August 2005; 70–1
  - Rules of engagement. *BMJ: Career Focus.* 13 August 2005; 72
  - General practice – the bigger picture. *BMJ: Career Focus.* 13 August 2005; 74
  - Dealing with rejection. *BMJ: Career Focus.* 13 August 2005; 75
  - More than an interview to land the job. *BMJ: Career Focus.* 13 August 2005; 78
  - Amos J-A. *Handling Tough Job Interviews.* Oxford: How To Books; 2007 and Corfield R. *Successful Interview Skills.* London: Kogan Page; 2006 were recommended.

Curriculum vitae

Try these sites for advice:
➤ www.careerslab.com/
➤ www.medical-interviews.co.uk/default.aspx
➤ www.careers.lon.ac.uk/output/Page19.asp

See Ariyasena H, Tewari N and Livesley PJ. The search for the perfect curriculum vitae. *BMJ Career Focus.* 2005; **331**: 167–9.
Avoid the four 'bad' CV types:
1 the functional overkill
2 the too traditional
3 the aggressive modern
4 the template.

Primary care administration and IM&T

Health economics

The concepts of QALYs (quality adjusted life years) and HYEs (health year equivalents) can form the basis of a tutorial.

Management tools

Surveys have indicated that most trainees have only limited understanding of practice management at the end of the year.

Consider:

➤ going through last year's accounts with them (practice and personal)

➤ running a mock job application process at the end of the year selecting a practice from the BMJ, writing a mock letter of application, a reply and a mock interview (even a mock rejection!)

➤ show and discuss the practice agreement with the trainee

➤ try to give them a real area of responsibility, e.g. ordering some equipment, looking at the DDA system, etc.

E-mail tips

See Cooke M, Ballé SJ, Régnier A. Lean e-mail: applying the 6S to e-mail. *BMJ Careers Focus.* 20 Jan 2010.

1 Sweep
   ➤ Install a good spam filter.
   ➤ Do not ask for replies unless necessary.
   ➤ Use RSS feeds and personal blogs rather than journal alerts.
   ➤ Avoid broadcasting your e-mail address.
   ➤ Alot an 'e-mail check' time in your diary – avoid constant checking.
2 Sort
   ➤ Alot a dedicated time to get your e-mail account under control.
   ➤ Unsubscribe from unnecessary mailing lists.
   ➤ Create rules to filter out certain e-mails into specified folders, i.e. a read box.
3 Straighten
   ➤ Devise an effective e-filing system.
   ➤ Save e-mails to this and not the e-mail system.
4 Shine
   ➤ Tidy up every day.
   ➤ Set a target for your e-mail screen, i.e. only five left at each day end.
5 Systematise
   ➤ Be an efficient reader (*see* Chapter 8, Table 8.1).
   ➤ Be a good delegator (*see* Chapter 6).
   ➤ Encourage other users to be the same!

6   Sustain
> ➤ Have a system that works for you!
> ➤ Have a holiday plan.
> ➤ Remember the IT rules – particularly 'IT is NOT always the answer' – sometimes phones and even letters are better!
> ➤ Remember to update your IT skills.

Communication and consulting skills

BATHE and ICE

This is a simple reminder of how to inquire about possible psychological elements of a problem. It is useful for the 'medical model' trainee.
Ask about:

Background	What is happening in your life currently?
Affect	How do you feel?
Troubles	Is anything worrying you at the moment?
Handling	How are you managing at the moment?

Show:

Empathy	That sounds hard. It must be difficult.

The ice simply adds:

Ideas	Why do you think this has happened?
Concerns	Have you any other questions? and
Expectations	What can we do about this?

Chunk, chop, check

This is a brief reminder of how to share information. Put the information into related **chunks** or blocks, **chop** these into bite sized short sentences, and **check** where they have gone – ask the patient!

PLISSIT

This is a counselling aide-memoir to act as a guide for the GP 'amateur' counsellor.

P	Permission from the patient for the doctor to adopt this role is often implied but really should be considered carefully by the doctor.
LI	The giving of Limited amounts of Information is appropriate
SS	The doctor should carefully consider any Specific Suggestions that they may consider, i.e. are they appropriate?
IT	The doctor should consider whether this patient needs Intensive Treatment, i.e. referral should be considered.

Prevention: the 'Stages of Change Model'

See Prochaska S and Diclemente C. Towards a comprehensive model of change. In: Miller W and Heather N, editors. *Treating Addictive Behaviour: processes of change*. New York: Plenum Press; 1986. This is a five-stage model to help link prevention activity to the patient's motivational stage.

Stage 1   Pre-contemplation: raise awareness by feeding back the patient's views, aiming to produce cognitive dissonance (i.e. make them uncomfortably aware).

Stage 2   Contemplative: reflect positive statements and encourage solutions for change.

Stage 3   Action: provide information, choices, goal setting, active support.

Stage 4   Maintenance: provide follow-up (personal, group, community, etc.). Reinforce behaviours, outcomes and strategies to prevent relapse.

Stage 5   Relapse: analyse reasons for relapse, support and encourage.

Prevention: The '4A' model

This is a simple aide-memoir to encourage screening activity in the consultation. Remember to Ask Advise Assist and Arrange follow up. (from the RACGP)

Data gathering and interpretation

Kipling's six honest men

> I keep six honest serving men: they taught me all I know
> Their names are what and why and who, and where and when and how

This can be used to encourage a more analytical approach in the 'poetic'!

Evidence quality: the Canadian assessment scheme

This is a simple lettering scheme that grades the evidence-based reliability of the area looked at.

A   Good evidence available to support this action.

B   Fair evidence to support this action.

C   Equivocal or incomplete evidence to support this action.

D   Some evidence to suggest this action is not advisable.

E   Good evidence to suggest this action is not indicated.

An increasing number of publications are beginning to use this system to aid clinicians. It has been applied to screening procedures and drug use particularly.

Evidence quality: the SIGN system

A   At least one quality meta-analysis, systematic review of RCTs or RCT trial with a very low risk of bias and directly applicable to the target population. OR

A body of evidence consisting of principally of well-controlled meta-analyses, systematic reviews of RCTs, or RCTs with a low risk of bias directly applicable to the target population and demonstrating consistency of results.

B A body of evidence, including studies rated as high-quality systematic reviews of case-control or cohort studies, and high-quality case-control or cohort studies, with a very low risk of bias or confounding and a high probability that the relation is causal and which are directly applicable to the target population and with overall consistency of results. OR Extrapolated from studies described in A.

C A body of evidence including well-conducted case-control or cohort studies with a low risk of confounding or bias and a moderate possibility that the relation is causal and which are directly applicable to the target population and with overall consistency of results. OR Extrapolated from studies described in B.

D Non-analytical studies, such as case reports, case series or expert opinion. OR Extrapolated from studies described in C.

Good Practice Points (GPP)

Recommended best practice based on clinical experience of the guideline development group.

'Tiering'

This is a technique used to increase a trainee's awareness of the rationale behind their behaviour in practice. It is also useful in preparation for the MRCGP. For a particular action the learner runs through the following tiered hierarchy, going as far down the tiers as they think necessary or possible.

Tier 1   What is your normal practice?
Tier 2   What is your peer group normal practice?
Tier 3   What are the current professional views in this area?
Tier 4   Is there a relevant consensus document or set of guidelines?
Tier 5   Is there published evidence of relevance?
Tier 6   Can you name the evidence?
Tier 7   Can you comment on the quality of the evidence?
Tier 8   Can you provide detail of the specific literature?

Making a diagnosis/making decisions

SOAP

This established system is useful for the trainee who has problems note keeping or structuring their thoughts.

Subjective: What did the patient say?
Objective: What evidence of ill health have I elicited?

Assessment: What do we make of the situation?

Plan: What are we going to do?

Threshold of diagnosis recognition graph

This is a concise way of illustrating the problems of diagnosis in general practice, i.e. different diseases look the same early on, need different levels of safety netting depending on their pattern of progression and the threshold of presentation and recognition varies from person to person and doctor to doctor, i.e. life's a bitch! (*See* Figure 9.1.)

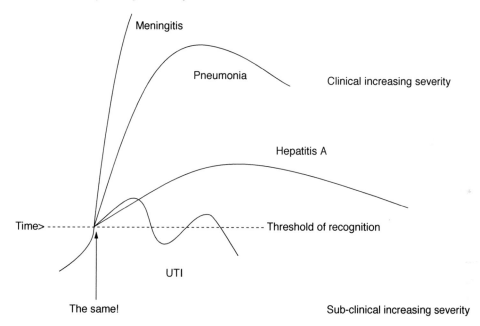

Figure 9.1 Threshold of diagnosis recognition graph

Managing medical complexity

Heartsink patients

The four categories of heartsink patients can form the basis of an interesting tutorial – particularly with the added concept that it may be heartsink doctors who get heartsink patients.

1 Manipulative help rejecter.
2 Entitled demander.
3 Dependent clinger.
4 Self-destructive denier.

'Sieving'

This is a technique designed to increase awareness of the implications of primary care behaviours. It expands the horizons of the trainee and is useful

MRCGP preparation. The implications of a particular action are put through a series of 'sieves' to see if there are any potential effects. The sieves may vary from problem to problem. An example is shown in Table 9.2.

Table 9.2 Problem sieve

Patient's sieve	Doctor's sieve	Practice sieve	Management sieve	Other sieve
Patient	Doctor	Finance	Finance	Finance
Primary carers	Partners	Staff	Trusts	Drug companies
Families	Colleagues	PHCT	Secondary care	
Communities	Profession	Primary care groups	Health authority government	

Practising holistically

Prevention

Try this on your 'classical' trainee. Aesculapis had two daughters: Panacea (the goddess of cure) and Hygiena (the goddess of prevention). How do you think they related to each other and why? (They continually fought!) This can provide a stimulus for discussion about the tensions between curative and preventative medicine – nothing is new!

How to write a poem

Advice by Eileen Gunstone can form the basis of tutorials on many areas: *see* www.radcliffepublishing.com/gptrainershandbook and www.docstoc.com/docs/2683526/An-introduction-to-writing-poetry

Community orientation

➤ Run a tutorial based on a recent edition of the local paper.
➤ Identify local community groups and suggest trainee does a project/talk with them.

Maintaining an ethical approach

➤ Write some 'scenarios' that involve obvious ethical dilemmas.
➤ Base a tutorial around the various ethical models (i.e. four principles plus scope, utilitarianism, consequentialism, deontology . . .): perhaps for the theorist.
➤ Look at the relevant section of GMC documentation 'Good Medical Practice' 'Duties of a doctor'.

Fitness to practise

Stress at work

1 **The three 'Cs'**: if present, these reduce levels of stress:
   - Control
   - Commitment
   - Challenge.
2 **The three 'horizons'**: have three horizons to look at each with the promise of a positive experience, i.e. make plans that you look forward to in the short, intermediate and long-term future.
3 **The three 'times' table**: stress can be reduced by having time for:
   - oneself
   - a friend/mate
   - a group (not usually medical).
4 **Enjoy the now**
   - recognise that the only real time is now
   - the past is gone and the future is unpredictable
   - look for satisfaction in every situation and now.
5 **Know yourself:** if you can achieve this, you can manage your own resources to better effect.
   - Know you moods.
   - Know your personality.
   - Know your transferences (i.e. feelings that dredge up hidden meanings).
   - Know your 'gotchas' (i.e. actions/situations/words that get to you).
   - Know your agendas (i.e. what you want).
   - Know your current stress level.
   - Know your actual communication skill level.
   - Know you visionary dust depth (how long is it since you dusted your dreams?).
   - Know when to get help.
6 **The 'ten commandments' of stress reduction**
   - Thou shalt **not** be perfect or even try to be.
   - Thou shalt **not** try to be all things to all people.
   - Thou shalt leave things undone which ought to have been done.
   - Thou shalt **not** spread thyself too thin.
   - Thou shalt learn to say **NO**.
   - Thou shalt **not** feel guilty.
   - Thou shalt schedule time for thyself and thy friends.
   - Thou shalt switch off and do nothing regularly.
   - Thou shalt be boring, untidy, inelegant and unattractive at times.
   - Thou shalt be thine own best friend and **never** thine own worst enemy.

Maintaining performance: learning and teaching

Assumptions

This a useful way of challenging a trainee who makes assumptions inappropriately. Write down the word assume and then divide it as shown: ASS/U/ME, i.e. assume makes an ASS out of U and ME!

Disney theory

Walt Disney apparently had three rooms which he used to develop his cartoons. The 'Dream' room where any ideas were allowed with no restraint (i.e. everything is possible). The 'Solution' room where answers to each problem were considered assuming limitless resources (i.e. all problems have solutions). Finally, the 'Reality' room, where a product must emerge. These states can be used to consider problems and help by encouraging breadth of thought and dropping the baggage of past restraints. *See* for more details: www. trulyhumancoaching.com/neurolinguistic_programming_articles/disney_creative_strategy.pdf

Juggling

At some stage in the year, the trainee has to face choices. Making choices often involves dropping options. An interesting way of exploring this is to use a set of juggling balls with labels for the choices. As a particular choice is literally dropped the trainees' feelings can be explored. Even good jugglers can be made to drop the ball!

The 'virtual' surgery

All trainers are familiar with random case analysis and selective case analysis. An interesting variation is to write a brief 'virtual' surgery list covering the area of your tutorial theme, i.e. if you are looking at asthma write brief presentations for about 10 patients covering the points you feel relevant/ difficult.

NESCAFE

This is a pneumonic to encourage critical prescribing.
- Is the drug   Necessary?
- Is the drug   Effective?
- Is the drug   Safe?
- Is the drug   Cost-effective?
- Are there any   Alternatives?
- What   Follow up is indicated?
- Does the drug have any   Extra features?

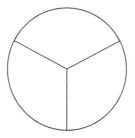

COGNITIVE
Acquire and use
relevant knowledge

AFFECTIVE
Acquire and use relevant
interpersonal and relationship
behaviours and feelings

PSYCHOMOTOR
Acquire the relevant neuromuscular skills

Figure 9.2 Patient problem pie

Patient problem pie
This is a system for analysing the possible learning requirements generated by a patient presentation. The trainee is encouraged to produce a breakdown of the skills and knowledge required to tackle the problem using three areas: cognitive, affective and psychomotor. The constituent elements of each of these areas are analysed and learning needs derived from this. The 'pie' is illustrated in Figure 9.2.

Props and stunts
➤ Change the tutorial environment: go for a walk!
➤ Show some pictures: Michelangelo's 'Pieta' to illustrate releasing the inner learner, Escher's work to discuss perspectives; Dali's work to talk about time, space and stress; Constable to illustrate tranquillity, etc.
➤ Use some poetry or quotations, etc., etc.

Planning a teaching session – acronym 'AOMREF'
➤ Aims   Where are heading?
➤ Objectives   How will we know we are there?
➤ Methods   How are we going to get there?
➤ Resources   What do we need for the trip?
➤ Evaluation   Where are we?
➤ Follow-up   What does the learner need to do next

The seven habits of highly effective people
See Covey SR. *The 7 Habits of Highly Effective People: powerful lessons in personal change.* London: Simon & Schuster Ltd; 2000. This site (www.franklincovey. com/tc/mediaengine/public/files/art_seven_habits_revisited.pdf) has a nice

(short) summary of this book – the principles can form the basis of a tutorial around developing good intra- and interpersonal skills. The site contains a lot of other potential resources based on the model.

Ethical models

Trainers mentioned a number of these models that can be used in tutorials to widen trainee's awareness:

1   Four principles plus scope (Gillon R. Medical ethics: four principles plus attention to scope. *BMJ.* 1994; **309**: 184–8): the best-known model using the following categories:
    (a)   Autonomy, Confidentiality, Consent and Communication.
    (b)   Maleficence: do not harm.
    (c)   Beneficence: do some good.
    (d)   Justice: legal, moral, resource and natural.
    The main criticism of this model is that is does not help you define which principles may take precedence.
2   Utilitarianism: in summary, 'the greatest good for the greatest number' – perhaps arguably 'the ends justify the means'?
3   Deontology: in summary an ethical theory based on doing the 'right' things according to rules, duty or obligation. Arguably, 'the means justify the ends'?
4   DISORDER: a system that can help define how to resolve an ethical dilemma:
    ➤ Define the dilemma.
    ➤ Inquiry for information.
    ➤ Sorting out who are the stakeholders.
    ➤ Options and Outcomes.
    ➤ Rights and Rules.
    ➤ Determination of decision.
    ➤ Evaluation of effects.
    ➤ Review and Reconsideration.

Audit

➤ *See* at: www.radcliffepublishing.com/gptrainershandbook for the one-page guide to audit.
➤ Look on the Dundee site – possibly the longest list of potential audits you'll ever find! – at: www.dundee.ac.uk/gptraining/summative/AuditTitles.htm
➤ Other useful sites for audit www.clinicalauditsupport.com/what_is_clinical_audit.html; http://mypimd.ncl.ac.uk/ecvts/green-book/audit/some-ideas-for-audits and www.clinicalgovernance.scot.nhs.uk/.../ideasforauditandSEA.rtf

SUMMARY

This list could probably be endless. It illustrates the breadth and depth of approach trainers use. These approaches will continue to multiply and evolve to the benefit of the trainees. This is probably best summed up by two comments trainers made on the 1998 questionnaire:

➤ 'I'm not sure if I'm a good trainer but I think I'm a good educational resource.'

➤ 'I have never got it quite right: is this the challenge or am I just crap?'

CHAPTER 10

Quality issues: how am I driving?

Okay, so this is a poor effort at making an interesting title about evaluating your own performance as a trainer and a training practice. 'Oh no!', I hear you cry.

> How do you assess the quality of training/tutorials you provide?

This was one of the questions posed in our survey of GP trainers. One of the responses was:

> I know I should – how do others?

Ten points for honesty. Maybe we should take one step back and change this to 'WHY should I evaluate my own teaching methods?'

WHY EVALUATE YOUR TEACHING?

There is a trend from the questionnaire responses that evaluation is happening less often. Therefore, simply telling you that it is a 'good thing' to do does not seem adequate. Let's divide this into two sections based on the concept of 'motivation'. Mohanna K, Wall D and Chambers R. *Teaching Made Easy: A Manual for Health Professionals*. Oxford: Radcliffe Medical Press; 2004, introduces the concept that motivation can be positive (e.g. inspired by others, deep interest in a subject) or negative (e.g. fear of adverse things happening if you don't do something). Positive motivation tends to lead to a deeper understanding.

Chapter 1 discusses the requirements of GP trainers. Part of these relate to your ongoing personal development. This will include having an up-to-date educational personal development plan and undergoing a performance review. The aim will be for trainers to be re-accredited every three years. This process will include observation of your own teaching. This in itself is a form of evaluation.

Before the introduction of the e-portfolio, there were often discussions within our trainers group about what happens when things go wrong. For example, a trainee who is not successful in their assessments then questions the quantity/quality of teaching provided by the trainer. With this in mind, trainers would often use the feedback forms from tutorials as both evaluation and a record of educational activity. Although this has been partially overtaken by the e-portfolio learning log (*see* Chapter 4), this only reflects the content of the educational activity, not necessarily then quality. Therefore, to some extent, you have to do this!

Seeking feedback can feel like yet another task to include in addition to your already very packed life. Some trainers feel that the only feedback that is of any relevance is that of the final assessment (i.e. MRCGP). Some would argue that we are in the process of providing the skills for lifelong learning and providing a safe and enjoyable learning environment. Passing the MRCGP does not necessarily mean that the above are true. Secondly, evaluation of our own teaching process is ongoing. In order to improve we need to be aware *where* we need to improve. If your past three trainees have not passed the MRCGP and you have to question your teaching methods, what evidence can you use in order to evaluate where to make changes?

So, now that you have been persuaded that it is worth thinking about, let's think about the how.

HOW CAN I EVALUATE THE TEACHING I PROVIDE?
This can be divided into environment (the practice), process (your and your colleagues' teaching) and assessment (the MRCGP).

The practice
Chapter 1 discussed the requirements for an approved training practice. The re-accreditation process, as discussed earlier in that chapter, will include ensuring the practice still meets the required standards.

Educational process
One of the limitations to obtaining feedback will be the learner's reluctance to give negative feedback to their own trainer. You are, after all, the person responsible for helping them progress to the next stage of their career. If you have given your trainee a one-to-one tutorial, you will struggle to find a way that you can make learner feedback anonymous! This can be partially overcome by including an end-of-attachment questionnaire for the trainee. By this time they will have (hopefully) passed their assessments and be in a position not to feel compromised by giving honest feedback. An example of such a questionnaire can be found at: www.gp-training.net/training/docs/tq.pdf

There are a number of methods by which you can obtain learner feedback. Techniques/evidence used by trainers include:
1 written feedback
2 verbal feedback

3 video of teaching session and reflection on this
4 discussion of current teaching methods at trainee workshops
5 rating scales for trainees to complete.

Regardless of what technique you employ, in order to make it useful you need to be clear on what you are evaluating. Kirkpatrick's hierarchy helps to define the depth to which you are seeking feedback (*see* Box 10.1).

BOX 10.1 *Hierarchy of evaluation*

Level 1 – Reaction   (participant satisfaction)
Level 2 – Learning   (knowledge and skills acquired)
Level 3 – Behaviour (putting this knowledge into practice)
Level 4 – Results   (does this transfer into the community)
(Adapted from Kirkpatrick DI. Evaluation of training. In: Craig R and Maittel I. *Training and Development Handbook*. London: McGraw Hill; 1967.)

In essence – if learners don't enjoy the process, they are less likely to learn, and learning new information is only part of the process. We want to know how it can change their practice. An example of how you can put this into practice in the form of a written questionnaire can be found at: www.radcliffepublishing.com/gptrainershandbook

The majority of these are looking at one episode of teaching. There are other tools available (such as the end of year assessment) that can be used to try and correlate the quality of the educational experience in a broader sense.

Assessment

Passing the MRCGP will always be the primary aim of the trainee (think back to Maslow –they will not be interested in the philosophy of general practice if they can't pass the exam and get a job). Potential trainees will also be very interested in previous trainees' performance.

SUMMARY

Although the statutory approval system should ensure a minimum quality of training, this process will only happen every three years. The process of improving and maintaining quality is ongoing. This chapter has aimed to highlight the significance of evaluating your own training along with ideas of how this can be achieved.

The trainer's tutorial assessment form

This form combines the elements of at least 15 individual forms in current use. It aims to serve a number of functions:
1   to act as record of the learning experience/tutorial
2   to act as a planning aid
3   to encourage feedback from the trainee and Clinical Supervisor.

A. SUBJECT AREA

B. AIMS/OBJECTIVES
1
2
3

C. DATE OF ACTIVITY AND METHODS EMPLOYED

D. TRAINEE COMMENTS
Please mark the scales as appropriate:

       very enjoyable   not very enjoyable

Enjoyment _____

Relevance _____

Use of method _____

Please comment on:
1. Were our objectives reached?
2. Has this session raised new objectives? (with description)
3. Any other comments at all?

E. SUPERVISOR NAME
Supervisor comments: particularly on areas for development and comments relevant to this trainee and relationship to e-portfolio.

PLEASE RETURN THIS FORM TO THE TRAINEE
(The trainee must arrange for the trainer to receive a photocopy)

THANK YOU

The assessor's tutorial assessment form

This is an amalgamation of at least three forms currently available for assessing tutorials. Generally they are applied after observing a tutorial (sitting in, video or role play).

They have been used in trainers workshops to look at tutorial skills.

TUTORIAL ASSESSMENT FORM

Competence	*Exemplary*	*5*	*4*	*3*	*2*	*1*	*Poor Comment*

1 Preparation
2 Environment
3 Communication
    (and baggage check)
4 Relationship
5 Learner-centred
    - assessing needs
    - setting aims
    - choosing method
6 Appropriate structure
    - time
    - method
    - develops trainees
      self-awareness
    - develops trainee
    critical thinking
7 Flexibility
8 Evaluation
    - by trainee
    - by trainer
9 Future planning
10 Use of Curriculum
    and e-portfolio

Tutorial evaluation: 'KISS' (Keeping It Short and Simple)

Date:

Trainer:

Trainee:

Intended outcomes for the tutorial:

WHAT WENT WELL TODAY?

WHAT GOT IN THE WAY OF LEARNING?

WHAT COULD HAVE BEEN DONE DIFFERENTLY?

WHAT WILL CHANGE AS A RESULT OF THE TUTORIAL?

Assessment of trainer's performance: random case analysis

A. PROCESS

1	Case selection is random	⊔⊔⊔⊔⊔⊔	Case selection is influenced by the trainer or trainee.
2	The trainer/trainee dominates discussions.	⊔⊔⊔⊔⊔⊔	The discussion are balanced
3	Lack of respect for trainee's knowledge, values, feelings.	⊔⊔⊔⊔⊔⊔	Shows respect for trainee's knowledge. values, feelings.

B. AMBIENCE

1	No interruptions.	⊔⊔⊔⊔⊔⊔	Frequent interruptions.
2	Setting is uncomfortable and tense.	⊔⊔⊔⊔⊔⊔	Setting is comfortable and relaxed.
3	Poor use of eye contact.		Uses eye contact appropriately.

C. EVALUATION OF TEACHING SKILLS

1	Overuse of closed or rhetorical questions. Tends to be didactic.	⊔⊔⊔⊔⊔⊔	Uses open/reflective questions. Encourages learner to discover own solution.
2	Appears rushed, pressure to complete task.	⊔⊔⊔⊔⊔⊔	Unhurried, appropriate use of silence, prepared to listen.
3	Responds to verbal/non verbal cues. Flexible agenda.	⊔⊔⊔⊔⊔⊔	Ignores cues, sticks rigidly to agenda.
4	The trainer uses a challenging/ probing approach.	⊔⊔⊔⊔⊔⊔	The trainer colludes in avoiding difficult issues.
5	Tends to be destructive/ supportive.	⊔⊔⊔⊔⊔⊔	Attempts to build confidence.
6	The trainer shows appropriate recognition of trainee's needs.	⊔⊔⊔⊔⊔⊔	The trainer fails to show appropriate recognition of the trainee's needs.
7	The trainer does not recognise teaching opportunity.	⊔⊔⊔⊔⊔⊔	The trainer recognises opportunity for teaching.

D. FEEDBACK

1	The teacher does not provide constructive feedback.	⊔⊔⊔⊔⊔⊔	The teacher provides constructive feedback.
2.	No summary.	⊔⊔⊔⊔⊔⊔	The teacher is able to summarise.
3.	Areas or strengths and weaknesses not shared.	⊔⊔⊔⊔⊔⊔	The areas of strengths and weaknesses have been successfully shared.
4.	Opportunities for further development are identified.	⊔⊔⊔⊔⊔⊔	Opportunities for further study not identified.

CHAPTER 11

The 'difficult' trainee: how do trainers deal with challenging trainees?

Difficult: not easy; hard to perform; obscure; involved; hard to get on with; troublesome; stubborn (Penguin English Dictionary)

INTRODUCTION

It has been repeatedly stated throughout this book that taking on a GP trainee can be one of the most rewarding experiences of you career. Trainers are motivated by various factors including the challenge of training, the stimulation and the ultimate reward of seeing your trainee 'grow' and qualify in their own right. However, not every experience can be a smooth ride.

Encountering problematic trainees can leave you feeling drained, frustrated and disappointed. And this is only if you have managed to identify the problem in the first place. This chapter aims to give an overview of identifying potential problems, how to approach them and when and where to seek help. Most regional offices produce advice booklets and these should be read in conjunction with the following thoughts.

CAN WE PREDICT THE CHALLENGING TRAINEE?

Trainers have identified the following as markers for potential difficulty.

➤ Perceived lack of enthusiasm.
➤ Perceived lack of empathy.
➤ Long secondary care career (relating to an ingrained doctor-centred approach to consulting).
➤ Perceived tiredness.
➤ Attitudes about workload, e.g. study leave, holidays.
➤ Career breaks.
➤ Difficult 'life issues'.
➤ Language issues.
➤ International medical graduates (IMGs) (relating to linguistic, cultural and differences in educational/exam environments).

➤ Perceived 'professionalism' problems (the three Ts):
 – **Time** issues (late, disorganised, etc.)
 – **Task** issues (no follow-through, accepting responsibility)
 – **Thought** issues (i.e. attitude 'I don't need to do that', etc.).

Is should be remembered that none of these factors on its own guarantees that there will be problems, but the list should at least make you aware of potential difficulties.

Thoughts on international medical graduates (IMGs)

The vast majority of IMGs will be excellent trainees in their own right and the challenges they face are often related to the complexity of communication and cultural issues in primary care. Poor English skills are unusual and they will probably have been assessed using PLAB or IELTS. However, trainees may still struggle with local dialect or even rapidity of speech in stressful circumstances. Think back to how you felt dealing with your first few patients in general practice: now imagine doing it in a second language in another country! As ever, seek first to understand and don't be afraid to explore these issue with the trainee. It may also be worth seeking out trainers with previous or current experience of IMGs,

How do challenging trainees present?

Although there will be some overlap with markers of *potential* difficulty, the following is a list of how problematic trainees have *presented*.
➤ Over-confident trainees.
➤ The trainee who is always right (unable to compromise).
➤ Trainees with poor English language skills.
➤ Trainees with rigid, fixed belief systems.
➤ Abrasive trainees (usually reported by the staff).
➤ Very shy trainees.
➤ Clinically incompetent trainees.
➤ Trainees with exceptionally poor communication skills.
➤ The 'reluctant' trainee, i.e. simply doing time with no drive or enthusiasm.
➤ The 'distracted' trainee, i.e. one with severe outside pressures.
➤ The 'unhappy' trainee, i.e. away from home, family, etc.
➤ The 'unaware' trainee, i.e. no personal insight.
➤ The trainee with a drug problem.
➤ The excellent trainee who challenges and extends the trainer.
➤ The indecisive trainee.
➤ The impaired trainee (mental or severe physical impairment).
➤ The 'business' trainee, i.e. has other business-type commitments.
➤ The 'odd' or ' angry' trainee.

Problems can also be categorised in terms of good old 'knowledge, skills and attitudes' (*see* Table 11.1)

Table 11.1 Potential problem areas

Knowledge	Skills	Attitudes
Prescribing	Communication	I'm the doctor
Emergencies	Consulting	I'm qualified now
Surgery protocols	Practical, e.g. minor surgery, self-education	Time-keeping
Team roles		Preparation
QOF		On call
		Availability
		Dress
		Behaviour
		Flexibility re workload
		Self-confidence
		Motivation
		Organisation
		Delegation

This is taken from a very helpful section on the gp-training website, for more information go to: www.gp-training.net/training/educational_theory/difficulties/index.htm

It has already been mentioned that many deaneries will produce their own booklet relating to trainees in difficulty. These are often more helpful in relation to 'doing things by the book', e.g. for sickness, conduct issues, etc. They will often divide trainee problems into the following main areas.

➤ Personal conduct.
➤ Professional conduct.
➤ Competence and performance issues.
➤ Health and sickness issues.

Examples of deanery publications can be found at: www.westmidlandsdeanery. nhs.uk/Home/Publications.aspx and www.eastmidlandsdeanery.nhs.uk/ document_store/12547568061_managing_performance_problems_-_gp_ specialty_registrars.pdf

HOW DO I APPROACH THE PROBLEMATIC TRAINEE?

> The biggest trainer problem we find is lack of documentation. (Region)
> The biggest and most difficult trainee problem is lack of insight. (Region)

This is taken from a paper written for the West Midlands deanery in 2003 (at: www.bradfordvts.co.uk/ONLINERESOURCES/03.7%20TEACHING%20

AND%20LEARNING%20-%20esp%20good%20for%20Trainers/DIFFICULT
%20TRAINEES/doctors%20in%20difficult%20-%20WM%20deanery%20
guidance.doc) which includes some useful thoughts on the general approach,
these include the following.

➤ Tackle problems when they occur – do not leave it all to the end of the
  job.
➤ Find out the facts – there are at least two sides to everything.
➤ Share the problem with others – ask for help at an early stage
➤ Document everything that you do.
➤ Explain the problem constructively – set realistic targets and measure
  success.

If you as the trainer have either identified a problem with the trainee, or one
has been brought to your attention – act on it. The following questions can be
helpful in defining the nature of the problem.

➤ What is the problem?
➤ Who is it a problem for?
➤ What is the effect of the problem?
➤ Am I prepared to put up with the problem?
➤ Does the trainee accept there is a problem?
➤ Is there an underlying reason for the problem?
➤ What changes are we trying to negotiate?
➤ What are the consequences if changes agreed?
➤ What are the consequences if changes not agreed?
➤ What options are there for addressing the problem?
➤ Which is the best option?
➤ Who should deal with the problem?
➤ Does this create a knock-on problem?
➤ Is the trainee happy with the outcome?
➤ Spell out the consequences.
➤ How can the resolution be monitored?

Although this helps to structure your approach, it is also helpful to bear in
mind the following to facilitate the conversation.

➤ Be specific, use examples.
➤ Address the problem not the person.
➤ Express your feelings about the behaviour.
➤ Allow discussion.
➤ Let the trainee suggest solutions.
➤ Appropriate time, place, setting.
➤ Don't use humour.
➤ Summarise.

➤ Spell out consequences.
➤ Arrange follow-up.
➤ Look for hidden issues.

Most information relating to problematic trainee comes back to two recurring thoughts – act soon, and document everything! Remember, you are aiming to produce insight into the problems and a long-term outcome. You must also accept that change is solely in the power of the trainee.

As ever, the Bradford VTS website has some excellent resources relating to this at: www.bradfordvts.co.uk/PICKAPAGE/TRAINEESDIFFICULTY/difficult Trainee.htm

WHO SHOULD BE INFORMED, AND WHEN?

Most trainers feel that the local programme directors (formerly course organisers) should be notified sooner rather than later. Although they may not have significant input initially they will be able to give advice on your approach and when further intervention may be merited.

Should there be serious concerns over personal or professional conduct, this will usually progress from the programme directors to deanery involvement. In the most serious cases you may even have involvement with the GMC.

Any health issues identified must be approached from occupational health and encouraging the trainee to register with their local GP. Remember, you are NOT their doctor!

WHAT DO I DOCUMENT AND WHERE?

Prior to the e-portfolio, trainers would keep a folder of evidence and keep a written record of conversations relating to problems. These could be kept if needed as evidence of their efforts to address problems during training. Now that we have the e-portfolio, we reach a dilemma. Although this seems the most appropriate place to document discussions/concerns and long-term aims/outcomes, will it adversely affect your relationship with the trainee? Ultimately, the e-portfolio is a reflection of the trainee's progress through training. With this in mind, most trainers would feel that all problems and approaches should be noted as a record of the training process and also to avoid the risk of collusion with the trainee.

WHAT ABOUT ME?

There is a thought that if you have a large number of 'Heartsink' patients you ought to be looking at your own health, i.e. have you become the heartsink?

Problems with trainees can be draining, emotionally and physically. There-fore don't do it alone! Involve other members of the practice in the process and decisions. This is also where the local trainers group can be invaluable. Apart from supporting you through these difficult times it can also be an invaluable resource for ideas of who to inform and approaches to the problem.

SUMMARY

Problematic trainees can be a draining experience, both physically and emo-tionally. It is important to act soon, and have clear documentation. Many of these issues can be worked through between the trainee and trainer, and although this can be quite demanding, the outcome can be a real high point in training. Always be aware of the effect this has on you, obtain support from others and take the opportunity to reflect on your own practice and approach for future trainees.

References

There is a distinction between the references listed here (which the authors have referred to) and those listed in the text (which other Trainers have mentioned as useful). Readers should be aware of this.

Al-Shehri A. Learning by reflection. *Education for General Practice*. 1995; 7: 237–48.

Balint M. *The Doctor, His Patient and the Illness*. London: Pitman Medical; 1957.

Balint E and Norell J. *Six Minutes for the Patient*. London: Tavistock Press; 1973.

McCarthy B. *The Hemispheric Mode Indicator: right and left brain approaches to learning*. Barrington, IL: Excel; 1993.

Barrow H and Tamblyn R. *Problem-Based Learning: An approach to medical education*. New York, NY: Springer; 1980.

Battles JB, Dowell D L, Kirk M *et al*. The affective attributes of the ideal primary care specialist. In: Bender W *et al.*, editors. *Teaching and Assessing Clinical Competence*. Groningen: Boek Werk Publications; 1990.

Belbin R. *Management Teams: why they succeed or fail*. London: Heinemann; 1981.

Berne E. *Games People Play*. London: Penguin Books; 1977.

Biggs J. *Teaching for Quality Learning at University*. 2nd ed. Buckingham: Society for Research into Higher Education and Open University Press; 2003.

Blanchard KH. *Leadership and the One Minute Manager*. New York: Free Press; 1982.

Bligh J. The S-SDRLS: a short questionnaire about self directed learning. *Education for General Practice*. 1993; 4: 121–5.

Bligh J. Independent learning among GP trainees: an initial survey. *Medical Education*. 1992; 26: 497–50.

Brown G and Atkins M. *Effective Teaching in Higher Education*. London: Methuen; 1988.

Brown H. Becoming a General Practice Trainer. *BMJ*. 1999; **318**.

Burnard P. *Teaching Interpersonal Skills*. London: Chapman and Hall; 1991.

Byrne B and Long P. *Doctors Talking to Patients*. London: RCGP; 1976.

Campion P *et al*. *Teaching Medicine in the Community*. Oxford: Oxford University Press; 1997.

Coulson R and Osborne C. Ensuring curricular content in a student-directed problem-based learning program. In: Schmidt H and de Volder M, editors. *Tutorials in Problem-Based Learning*. The Netherlands: Van Gorcum and Co; 1984.

Cox K and Ewan C. *The Medical Teacher*. London: Churchill Livingstone; 1988.

Dunn A. Personal construct analysis. *Education for General Practice*. 1993; **2**: 121–25

Fabb W. *Proceedings of the Educational Symposium*. WONCA; 1997.

Fabb W *et al*. *Focus on Learning*. London: RCGP Family Medicine Programme. Beavergroup; 1976.

Foulkes F and Fulton P. Critical appraisal of published literature. *BMJ*. 1991; **302**: 1136.

Freeling P and Browne K. *The Doctor Patient Relationship*. London: Churchill Livingstone; 1976.

Fry J. *The Future General Practitioner*. London: RCGP; 1972

Glasser W. *Reality Therapy*. London: Harper and Row; 1965.

Guilbert J. *Education Handbook for Health Personnel*. 6th ed. Geneva: WHO (Offset Publication No 35); 1997.

Hall. A. *GP Trainers Handbook*. Oxford: Blackwell Scientific Press; 1983.

Harden R *et al*. The continuum of problem based learning. *Medical Teacher*. 1998; **20**: 317.

Harris T. *I'm OK You're OK*. London: Pan Books; 1973.

Havelock P, Hasler J, Flew R *et al*. *Professional Education for General Practice*. Oxford: Oxford University Press (Oxford General Practice series 31); 1997.

Helman CG. 'Feed a cold – starve a fever': folk models of infection in an English suburban community, and their relations to medical treatment. *Culture, Medicine and Psychiatry*. 1978; **2**(2): 107–37.

Helman D. Disease versus illness in general practice. *JRCGP*. 1981; **31**: 548–53.

Heron J. *Six Category Intervention Analysis. Human Potential Research Project*. Guildford: University of Surrey; 1986.

Honey P and Mumford A. *The Manual of Learning Styles*. Peter Honey: Maidenhead; 1992.

Howard. J. The emotional diary: a framework for reflective learning. *Education for General Practice*. 1997; **8**: 288–91.

Irby D. Teaching when time is limited. *BMJ*. 2008; **336**: 384.

Irby D. *Academic Medicine*. 1992; **67**(10): 630–8.

ICGP Time management: key ideas. In: *Handbook and Diary*. Dublin: ICGP; 1991.

Jarvis P. *The Theory and Practice of Teaching*. London: Kogan Page; 2002.

JCGPT. *Training for General Practice*. London: JCGPT; 1992.

JCGPT. *Accreditation of Regions and Schemes for Vocational Training in General Practice: general guidance*. London: JCGPT; 1992.

Jensen E. *Superteaching: turning points for teachers*. Barron's educational series; 1994.

Kelly AV. *The Curriculum. Theory and Practice*. 4th ed. London: Paul Chapman; 1999.

Kirkpatrick DI. Evaluation of training. In: Craig R and Maittel I. *Training and Development Handbook*. London: McGraw Hill; 1967.

Knowles M. *Self-directed Learning: a guide for learners and teachers*. New York, NY: Association Press; 1973.

Kolb D. *Experiential Learning: Experience at the source of learning and development*. Englewood Cliffs, NJ: Prentice Hall; 1984.

Landsberg M. *The Tao of Coaching*. Santa Monica, CA: Knowledge Exchange; 1997.

Levenstein J *et al*. The patient-centred clinical method. 1. A model for the doctor–patient interaction in family medicine. *Family Practice*. 1986; **3**(1): 24–30.

Lublin J. Role modelling: a case study in general practice. *Medical Education*. 1992; **26**: 116–22.

Macauley D. READER: an acronym for critical appraisal. *BJGP*. 1994; **44**: 83–5.

MacWhinney IR. Problem-solving and decision-making in primary medical practice. *Canadian Family Physician*. 1972; **18**: 109.

Maslow AH. *Motivation and Personality*. New York, NY: Harper and Row; 1972.

McEvoy P. *Educating the Future GP*. Oxford: Radcliffe Medical Press; 1993.

Miller *et al*. Motivation to learn. *BJGP*. 1998; **48**(432): 1430.

Mohanna K, Wall D and Chambers R. *Teaching Made Easy: a manual for health professionals*. Oxford: Radcliffe Medical Press; 2004.

Murtagh J. *General Practice*. 4th ed. Sydney: McGraw Hill; 1998.

Myerscough P and Ford J, editors. *Talking with Patients*. Oxford: Oxford Medical Publications; 1996.

Neame L. Problem orientated learning in medical education. In: Schmidt HG and De Volder ML, editors. *Tutorials in Problem-based Learning: a new direction in teaching the health professions*. The Netherlands: Van Gorcum; 1984.

Neighbour R. *The Inner Apprentice: an awareness-centred approach to. vocational training for general practice*. Dordrecht: Kluwer Academic; 1987, 1993.

Neighbour R. *The Inner Consultation: how to develop an effective and intuitive consulting style*. Lancaster: Kluwer Academic; 1987.

O'Connor J and Seymour J. *Introducing Neuro-linguistic Programming*. London: Aquarian Press; 1993.

Pendleton D, Schofield T, Havelock P and Tate P. *The Consultation: an approach to learning and teaching*. Oxford: Oxford University Press; 1984.

Pitts J. Pathologies of 1:1 teaching. *Education for General Practice*. 1996; **7**: 118–22.

Quirk M. *How to Learn and Teach in Medical School*. Springfield, IL: Charles C Thomas; 1994.

RCGP. *Priority Objectives for General Practice Vocational Training*. Occasional Paper 30. London: RCGP; 1988.

RCGP. *Rating Scales for Vocational Training in General Practice*. Occasional Paper 40. London: RCGP; 1988.

RCGP. *A System of Training for General Practice.* 2nd ed. Occasional Paper 4. London: RCGP; 1979.

Riding R and Cheema I. Cognitive styles: an overview and integration. *Educational Psychology.* 1991; **11**: 193–215.

Riding R and Rayner S. *Cognitive Styles and Learning Strategies.* London: David Fulton Publishers; 1998.

Rose C. *Accelerated Learning.* Great Missenden: Topaz; 1985.

Ruscoe M. Assessment of the tutorial. *Education for General Practice.* 1994; 5: 260–8.

Sandars J and Baron R. *Learning General Practice: a structured approach for trainee GPs and trainers.* Knutsford: Pastest Books; 1991.

Schön D. *Educating the Reflective Practitioner: toward a new design for teaching and learning in the professions.* San Francisco, CA: Jossey-Bass; 1987.

Schutz W. *The Interpersonal Underworld.* Palo Alto, CA: Science and Behaviour Books; 1966.

Seedhouse D. Avoiding the myths: a pre-requisite for teaching ethics. *Education for General Practice.* 1992; 3: 117–24.

Silverman J, Draper J and Kurtz SM. *Skills for Communicating with Patients.* Oxford: Radcliffe Medical Press; 1998.

Silverman J, Draper J and Kurtz SM. *Teaching and Learning Communication Skills in Medicine.* Oxford: Radcliffe Medical Press; 1998.

Skrabenek P. *The Death of Humane Medicine and the Rise of Coercive Healthism.* London: Social Affairs Unit; 1994.

Stott N and Davis R. The exceptional potential in each primary care consultation. *JRCGP.* 1979; **66**: 201–5.

Strasser R. How we teach key aspects of general practice. *Medical Teacher.* 1991; 1: 93.

Stewart MR and Lieberman III JA. *The 15-Minute Hour: Applied psychotherapy for the primary care physician.* 2nd ed. Westport, CT: Praegar; 1993.

Tate P. *The Doctor's Communication Handbook.* 6th ed. Oxford: Radcliffe Publishing; 2010; first published 1994.

Tudor Hart J. *A New Kind of Doctor.* London: Merlin Press; 1989.

Turner J *et al.* Assessment of trainer performance in RCA. *Education for General Practice.* 1998; 9: 99–202.

Index